Introduction

Welcome to "Old Fashioned Home Remedies - Combating the Common Cold with Amazing Results." In a world dominated by modern medicine, it's easy to overlook the incredible healing power of nature and the wisdom passed down through generations. This book takes you on a journey back to a time when simple, natural remedies were trusted allies in the battle against the common cold.

Though seemingly harmless, the common cold can leave us feeling miserable and drained. Sneezing, coughing, congestion, and fatigue can disrupt our daily lives and hinder our productivity. While over-the-counter medications provide temporary relief but often have unwanted side effects.

But fear not! Within the pages of this book, you'll discover a treasure trove of time-honored remedies that have withstood the test of time. These old-fashioned remedies offer relief from cold symptoms and strengthen your immune system, helping you combat future bouts of the common cold.

In our modern era, where convenience often trumps tradition, it's easy to forget the potent healing properties of herbs, spices, and other natural ingredients found in our kitchens and gardens. This book serves as a gentle reminder of the astonishing results that can be achieved by harnessing the power of nature.

Each chapter of this book delves into a specific aspect of combating the common cold. From herbal remedies and healing soups to steam therapy and essential oils, we explore a wide array of approaches that have stood the test of time. Additionally, we address the importance of rest, sleep, and a healthy lifestyle in bolstering your body's defenses against colds.

Remember, these remedies are not meant to replace professional medical advice. If you have underlying health conditions or your symptoms persist, it's always wise to consult a healthcare professional. However, for those seeking natural alternatives and a deeper connection to traditional wisdom, this book offers a wealth of knowledge and inspiration.

So, embark on this journey with an open mind and a willingness to embrace the remedies that have been trusted for generations. Say goodbye to the common cold and welcome the amazing results that await you within these pages. Get ready to unleash the power of old-fashioned home remedies and reclaim your health and vitality.

June 26, 2023

Chapter 1

Understanding the Common Cold

Section 1: Definition and Causes

The common cold, a frequent visitor in our lives, often catches us off guard with its unwelcome symptoms. In this section, we will explore the definition of the common cold and shed light on its causes, helping you gain a deeper understanding of this ubiquitous ailment.

Definition of the Common Cold: The common cold, also known as an upper respiratory tract infection, is a viral infection primarily affecting the nose and throat. It is characterized by a combination of symptoms such as a runny or stuffy nose, sneezing, coughing, sore throat, mild headache, and sometimes low-grade fever. Despite its name, the common cold is not caused by cold weather or exposure to chilly conditions but rather by a variety of viruses.

Causes of the Common Cold: Numerous viruses can cause the common cold, with rhinoviruses being the most prevalent culprits. Other common viral offenders include coronaviruses, adenoviruses, and respiratory syncytial viruses (RSV). These viruses are highly contagious and can spread from person to person through respiratory droplets expelled when an infected individual coughs, sneezes, or talks. Direct contact with contaminated surfaces or objects can also lead to viral transmission.

Understanding the causes of the common cold is crucial in implementing preventive measures and minimizing the risk of infection. By practicing good hygiene, such as regular handwashing, avoiding close contact with sick individuals, and maintaining a clean environment, you can significantly reduce your chances of catching a cold.

In the following sections, we will delve deeper into the symptoms, transmission, and prevention of the common cold, empowering you with knowledge to better navigate the challenges posed by this prevalent ailment. By understanding the enemy, we can arm ourselves with effective strategies to combat and overcome the common cold, paving the way for a healthier and more resilient future.
[End of Section 1]

Section 2: Common Symptoms

Recognizing the symptoms of the common cold is essential in differentiating it from other illnesses and seeking appropriate remedies. In this section, we will explore the typical signs and symptoms associated with the common cold, allowing you to identify and manage them effectively.

1. **Runny or Stuffy Nose**: One of the hallmark symptoms of the common cold is nasal congestion. You may experience a runny nose with clear or slightly colored mucus, or a stuffy nose that makes breathing through your nostrils difficult. This congestion is often accompanied by a feeling of pressure or heaviness in the sinuses.

2. **Sneezing**: Frequent bouts of sneezing are another common symptom of a cold. The irritation caused by the viral infection triggers the body's reflex to expel irritants, leading to repeated sneezing episodes.

3. **Coughing**: A persistent, dry cough is often present during a cold. It may be triggered by postnasal drip or irritation in the throat caused by the virus. While coughing is primarily a protective mechanism to clear the airways, it can be bothersome and may persist even after other symptoms subside.

4. **Sore Throat**: The throat may become sore, scratchy, or mildly painful due to inflammation caused by the viral infection. Swallowing and speaking may aggravate the discomfort, and you may notice a raw or scratchy sensation.

5. **Mild Headache**: Some individuals with a cold experience a mild headache or a feeling of pressure in the head. This is typically associated with sinus congestion and can vary in intensity.

6. **Fatigue and Malaise**: Feeling tired and lacking energy is common when you have a cold. The body's immune response and the viral infection

itself can contribute to a general sense of fatigue and malaise.

7. **Low-Grade Fever**: Although a fever is not a prominent feature of the common cold, some individuals may experience a low-grade fever, generally below 100.4°F (38°C). Fever is more commonly associated with other respiratory illnesses like the flu.

It's important to note that symptoms can vary from person to person, and their severity can range from mild to more pronounced. Additionally, certain symptoms, such as fever or severe headache, may indicate a different underlying condition requiring medical attention.

By familiarizing yourself with the common symptoms of a cold, you can take appropriate measures to manage them effectively and seek medical advice if needed. In the upcoming chapters, we will explore a wide range of old-fashioned home remedies to alleviate these symptoms and support your body's natural healing process.
[End of Section 2]

Section 3: Transmission and Prevention

Understanding how the common cold spreads and implementing preventive measures are vital in reducing the risk of infection and curtailing its transmission. In this section, we will explore the modes of transmission for the common cold and discuss effective strategies for prevention.

1. **Respiratory Droplets**: The primary mode of transmission for the common cold is through respiratory droplets. When an infected person

coughs, sneezes, or even talks, tiny droplets containing the cold virus are released into the air. These droplets can then be inhaled by nearby individuals, leading to infection.

2. **Direct Contact**: Direct contact with surfaces or objects contaminated with the cold virus can also facilitate its transmission. Touching your nose, mouth, or eyes after coming into contact with contaminated surfaces increases the risk of infection.

Preventive Measures:

a. Good Hygiene Practices:

- Wash your hands frequently with soap and water for at least 20 seconds, especially after being in public spaces, using the restroom, or touching surfaces that may be contaminated.
- If soap and water are not readily available, use hand sanitizers containing at least 60% alcohol.
- Avoid touching your face, particularly your nose, mouth, and eyes, to minimize the risk of transferring the virus from contaminated surfaces to your respiratory system.

b. Respiratory Etiquette:

- Cover your mouth and nose with a tissue or your elbow when coughing or sneezing to prevent respiratory droplets from dispersing into the air.
- Dispose of used tissues properly and wash your hands afterward.

c. Clean and Disinfect:

- Regularly clean and disinfect frequently touched surfaces, such as doorknobs, light switches, countertops, and electronic devices, using household disinfectants.

- Pay special attention to shared spaces and objects, such as kitchen and bathroom surfaces, telephones, and remote controls.

d. Avoid Close Contact:

- Minimize close contact with individuals who have a cold, and if possible, maintain a distance of at least six feet from them.
- If you have a cold, be considerate and avoid close contact with others to prevent spreading the virus.

e. Boost Your Immune System:

- Maintain a healthy lifestyle by eating a balanced diet, exercising regularly, and getting sufficient sleep to support your immune system's strength and resilience.

By implementing these preventive measures, you can significantly reduce the risk of contracting and spreading the common cold. Empower yourself with knowledge and adopt these practices as part of your daily routine to safeguard your health and the well-being of those around you.

In the subsequent chapters, we will explore an array of old-fashioned home remedies and lifestyle practices that can strengthen your immune system and provide relief from the common cold. By combining preventive measures with natural remedies, you can take proactive steps towards combatting the common cold and maintaining optimal health.

[End of Section 3]

Chapter 2

Strengthening Your Immune System

Section 1: Importance of a Strong Immune System

A robust immune system is essential for defending your body against various pathogens, including the viruses that cause the common cold. In this section, we will delve into the importance of having a strong immune system and how it plays a crucial role in preventing and fighting off illnesses.

1. **Defense Against Pathogens**: Your immune system acts as a complex network of cells, tissues, and organs that work together to recognize and eliminate harmful pathogens, such as viruses, bacteria, and fungi. A strong immune system is your body's first line of defense, constantly on guard to identify and neutralize potential threats before they can cause significant harm.

2. **Prevention of Infections**: A robust immune system plays a vital role in preventing infections. When your immune system is functioning optimally, it can identify and destroy invading

pathogens more efficiently, reducing the likelihood of falling ill. It acts as a protective shield, creating barriers and producing specialized cells and proteins that can recognize and target specific pathogens.

3. **Faster Recovery**: Even if an infection does occur, a strong immune system can significantly shorten the duration and severity of the illness. It mounts a rapid response, mobilizing immune cells and antibodies to combat the invading pathogens, thus aiding in a speedier recovery.

4. **Reduced Susceptibility to Infections**: Individuals with a weakened immune system are more vulnerable to infections, including the common cold. Certain factors, such as chronic stress, inadequate nutrition, lack of sleep, and underlying health conditions, can compromise the immune system's effectiveness. By strengthening your immune system, you can decrease your susceptibility to infections and enhance your overall well-being.

5. **Long-Term Health Benefits**: A strong immune system not only protects against acute illnesses but also offers long-term health benefits. Mounting evidence suggests that a healthy immune system is associated with a lower risk of chronic diseases, such as cardiovascular disease, diabetes, and certain types of cancer. By supporting your immune system, you can improve your overall health and quality of life.

Taking steps to strengthen your immune system is a proactive approach to maintaining optimal health and reducing the risk of infections, including the common cold. In the upcoming sections, we will explore various strategies, including nutritional tips and lifestyle practices, to boost and support your immune system naturally. By empowering your body's defense mechanisms, you can enhance your ability to ward off illnesses and enjoy a healthier, more resilient life.

Remember, while lifestyle factors can significantly influence your immune system, it is essential to consult with healthcare professionals for specific guidance, especially if you have underlying health conditions. Let's embark on this journey towards a stronger immune system and more vibrant well-being.
[End of Section 1]

Section 2: Nutritional Tips for Boosting Immunity

Proper nutrition plays a crucial role in supporting and strengthening your immune system. In this section, we will explore essential nutritional tips that can help boost your immune function and enhance your body's ability to ward off infections, including the common cold.

1. **Eat a Balanced Diet**: Aim for a well-rounded diet that includes a variety of nutrient-dense foods. Include ample amounts of fruits, vegetables, whole grains, lean proteins, and healthy fats in your meals. This provides your body with the necessary vitamins, minerals, antioxidants, and phytochemicals to support optimal immune function.

2. **Emphasize Antioxidant-Rich Foods**: Antioxidants help combat free radicals and oxidative stress, which can weaken the immune system. Incorporate foods rich in antioxidants, such as berries, citrus fruits, leafy greens, bell peppers, and nuts. These foods are packed with vitamins A,

C, and E, as well as other beneficial compounds that bolster immune health.

3. **Vitamin C**: Vitamin C is renowned for its immune-boosting properties. Include citrus fruits, berries, kiwi, broccoli, bell peppers, and leafy greens in your diet to ensure an adequate intake of vitamin C.

4. **Zinc**: Zinc is a mineral that plays a vital role in immune function. Include zinc-rich foods such as oysters, shellfish, lean meats, poultry, legumes, nuts, and seeds in your diet. If needed, consider zinc supplements under the guidance of a healthcare professional.

5. **Probiotics**: Probiotics are beneficial bacteria that promote a healthy gut microbiome, which is closely linked to immune function. Consume probiotic-rich foods like yogurt, kefir, sauerkraut, kimchi, and other fermented foods. Alternatively, consider probiotic supplements after consulting with a healthcare professional.

6. **Omega-3 Fatty Acids**: Omega-3 fatty acids have anti-inflammatory properties and support immune health. Include fatty fish (such as salmon, mackerel, and sardines), flaxseeds, chia seeds, walnuts, and avocados in your diet to ensure an adequate intake of these essential fats.

7. **Hydration**: Staying properly hydrated is crucial for optimal immune function. Drink an adequate amount of water throughout the day and incorporate hydrating foods like fruits, vegetables, herbal teas, and clear soups.

8. **Limit Processed Foods and Added Sugars**: Processed foods and excessive added sugars can contribute to inflammation and weaken immune function. Limit your intake of sugary beverages,

refined grains, and processed snacks. Opt for whole, unprocessed foods whenever possible.
Remember, a balanced diet rich in immune-boosting nutrients is just one piece of the puzzle. Other lifestyle factors, such as regular physical activity, sufficient sleep, stress management, and maintaining a healthy weight, also contribute to a strong immune system.

By adopting these nutritional tips and embracing a holistic approach to wellness, you can fortify your immune system, reducing your susceptibility to the common cold and other illnesses. In the subsequent chapters, we will explore additional lifestyle practices and natural remedies that further support immune health, allowing you to achieve optimal well-being and vitality.
[End of Section 2]

Section 3: Lifestyle Practices for Immune Support

In addition to a nutritious diet, certain lifestyle practices can significantly contribute to bolstering your immune system and supporting optimal health. In this section, we will explore key lifestyle practices that promote immune support and enhance your body's ability to defend against infections, including the common cold.

1. **Regular Physical Activity**: Engaging in regular exercise offers numerous benefits, including immune support. Moderate-intensity activities like brisk walking, jogging, cycling, or swimming can help improve circulation, reduce stress, and enhance the immune response. Aim for at least 150 minutes of moderate-intensity exercise per week, or as advised by your healthcare professional.

2. **Quality Sleep**: Adequate and restful sleep is vital for immune function. During sleep, your body repairs and rejuvenates itself, strengthening the immune system. Aim for 7 to 9 hours of uninterrupted sleep each night, creating a conducive sleep environment by maintaining a regular sleep schedule, keeping your bedroom dark and cool, and establishing a relaxing bedtime routine.

3. **Stress Management**: Chronic stress can weaken the immune system, making you more susceptible to infections. Explore stress management techniques that work for you, such as mindfulness meditation, deep breathing exercises, yoga, journaling, or engaging in hobbies and activities that bring you joy. Prioritize self-care and find healthy outlets to manage and reduce stress levels.

4. **Maintain a Healthy Weight**: Excess weight and obesity can negatively impact immune function. Strive to maintain a healthy weight through a balanced diet and regular physical activity. Consult with a healthcare professional or registered dietitian for personalized guidance and support in achieving your weight management goals.

5. **Hygiene Practices**: Practicing good hygiene habits is crucial for immune support and preventing the spread of infections. Wash your hands frequently with soap and water for at least 20 seconds, especially before eating, after using the restroom, and when returning home from public spaces. Avoid touching your face, particularly your eyes, nose, and mouth, to minimize the risk of introducing pathogens into your body.

6. **Stay Hydrated**: Proper hydration is essential for optimal immune function. Drink an adequate amount of water throughout the day to support the

transport of nutrients, elimination of toxins, and overall cellular function. Aim for at least 8 cups (64 ounces) of water daily, or adjust according to your body's needs and activity level.

7. **Limit Alcohol Consumption**: Excessive alcohol consumption can impair immune function. Moderate your alcohol intake or consider abstaining altogether to support your immune system and overall well-being.

By incorporating these lifestyle practices into your daily routine, you can provide your immune system with the support it needs to function optimally. Each small step contributes to strengthening your body's defenses and reducing the likelihood of falling ill, including from the common cold. In the following chapters, we will continue to explore natural remedies and strategies that further enhance immune support, empowering you to lead a healthier and more resilient life.

[End of Section 3]

Chapter 3

Herbal Remedies

Section 1: Echinacea - Nature's Immune Booster

Echinacea, a flowering plant native to North America, has been used for centuries as a natural remedy to support immune function. In this section, we will explore the benefits and uses of echinacea, shedding light on its role as a potent immune booster.

1. **Introduction to Echinacea**: Echinacea, also known as purple coneflower, is a herbaceous plant belonging to the daisy family. Its roots, flowers, and leaves are commonly used for medicinal purposes. Echinacea supplements are available in various forms, including capsules, extracts, and teas.

2. **Immune-Enhancing Properties**: Echinacea is renowned for its immune-enhancing properties. It contains a variety of active compounds, including flavonoids, alkamides, and polysaccharides, which stimulate the activity of immune cells, such as white blood cells. This immune-boosting action helps

your body's defense mechanisms respond more effectively to infections.

3. **Cold Prevention and Symptom Relief**: Echinacea has been traditionally used to prevent and alleviate symptoms of the common cold. Research suggests that echinacea can help reduce the severity and duration of cold symptoms, such as nasal congestion, sore throat, and cough. It may also help prevent recurrent respiratory infections when used as a preventive measure.

4. **Anti-Inflammatory and Antioxidant Effects**: In addition to its immune-enhancing properties, echinacea exhibits anti-inflammatory and antioxidant effects. These properties can help reduce inflammation, combat oxidative stress, and protect against cellular damage, further supporting immune health.

5. **Safe Usage and Considerations**: Echinacea is generally considered safe for short-term use in recommended dosages. However, it may interact with certain medications, such as immunosuppressants and medications metabolized by the liver. It is advisable to consult with a healthcare professional before using echinacea, especially if you have underlying health conditions or are taking medications.

6. **Forms and Dosage**: Echinacea is available in various forms, including liquid extracts, capsules, tablets, and teas. The appropriate dosage and duration of use may vary based on the specific product and individual needs. It is recommended to follow the manufacturer's instructions or seek guidance from a qualified herbalist or healthcare professional.

As with any herbal remedy, it is important to source high-quality echinacea products from reputable brands to ensure purity and potency. If you have any concerns or questions, consult with a healthcare professional before incorporating echinacea into your wellness routine.

Echinacea serves as a valuable tool in supporting immune health and preventing the common cold. However, it is just one piece of the herbal remedy puzzle. In the following sections, we will explore other herbal remedies that can provide relief and support for cold symptoms, empowering you to tap into the healing power of nature.
[End of Section 1]

Section 2: Ginger - A Warming Cold Remedy

Ginger, a versatile spice renowned for its distinct flavor and medicinal properties, has long been used as a natural remedy for various ailments, including the common cold.
In this section, we will delve into the warming benefits of ginger and its role in providing relief from cold symptoms.

1. **Warming Properties**: Ginger possesses warming properties that can help soothe the discomfort associated with cold symptoms. Its spicy and aromatic nature provides a comforting sensation, helping to alleviate congestion, promote circulation, and ease feelings of chilliness.

2. **Immune-Boosting Effects**: Ginger contains bioactive compounds, such as gingerol, which have potent antioxidant and anti-inflammatory properties. These compounds contribute to ginger's immune-boosting effects, supporting your body's natural defense mechanisms and enhancing its ability to fight off infections.

3. **Relieving Nasal Congestion**: Ginger is known to possess natural decongestant properties, making it beneficial for relieving nasal congestion. Consuming ginger or inhaling its steam can help clear blocked nasal passages, reduce mucus buildup, and ease breathing difficulties caused by a cold.

4. **Soothing Sore Throat and Cough**: Ginger's anti-inflammatory properties can help soothe a sore throat and calm coughing. Ginger tea or warm ginger-infused water with honey and lemon can provide relief by reducing throat irritation and suppressing coughing.

5. **Nausea Relief**: In addition to its effects on cold symptoms, ginger is also recognized for its ability to alleviate nausea and digestive discomfort. If a cold is accompanied by an upset stomach, consuming ginger in various forms, such as ginger tea or ginger candies, may help ease these symptoms.

6. **Ways to Incorporate Ginger**: There are multiple ways to incorporate ginger into your cold-fighting routine. You can brew ginger tea by steeping freshly grated ginger in hot water. Adding ginger to soups, stews, or stir-fries can infuse dishes with its distinct flavor and therapeutic benefits. Ginger supplements, available in capsule form, are also an option, but it is advisable to consult with a healthcare professional before adding them to your regimen.

As with any natural remedy, it's important to listen to your body and adjust the usage of ginger to suit your individual needs. If you have specific health conditions or concerns, it is recommended to consult with a healthcare professional before incorporating ginger into your routine.

Harness the warming and therapeutic power of ginger to alleviate cold symptoms and promote overall well-being. In the subsequent sections, we will explore additional herbal remedies that can provide relief and support during your battle against the common cold, allowing you to tap into the vast healing potential of nature.
[End of Section 2]

Section 3: Elderberry - The Immune-Enhancing Berry

Elderberry, a small dark purple fruit derived from the elder tree, has gained popularity for its immune-enhancing properties and potential benefits in fighting off colds and flu. In this section, we will explore the immune-boosting capabilities of elderberry and its role as a natural remedy for respiratory ailments.

1. **Immune-Boosting Effects**: Elderberry is rich in antioxidants and bioactive compounds, including anthocyanins and flavonoids, which contribute to its immune-enhancing effects. These compounds help support the immune system by reducing oxidative stress and inflammation, promoting a healthy immune response to infections.

2. **Cold and Flu Symptom Relief**: Elderberry has been traditionally used to alleviate symptoms of colds and flu. Studies suggest that elderberry may help reduce the duration and severity of respiratory symptoms, such as coughing, congestion, and sore throat. It may also aid in boosting recovery time from these illnesses.

3. **Antiviral Properties**: Elderberry exhibits antiviral properties, particularly against certain strains of the flu virus. Compounds found in elderberry can

interfere with the virus's ability to replicate and infect host cells, potentially reducing the severity and duration of flu symptoms.

4. **Anti-Inflammatory Benefits**: Inflammation plays a significant role in respiratory infections. Elderberry's anti-inflammatory properties can help reduce inflammation in the respiratory tract, providing relief from symptoms such as nasal congestion, cough, and sore throat.

5. **Forms and Dosage**: Elderberry is available in various forms, including syrups, extracts, capsules, and lozenges. It is important to follow the manufacturer's instructions or consult with a healthcare professional for appropriate dosage and usage guidelines. Elderberry products should come from reputable sources to ensure quality and safety.

6. **Safety Considerations**: While elderberry is generally safe for most individuals when used as directed, it is important to exercise caution. Raw or unripe elderberries contain certain compounds that can be toxic, so they should never be consumed without proper processing. Pregnant or breastfeeding women, individuals with autoimmune conditions, and those taking certain medications should consult with a healthcare professional before using elderberry.

Incorporating elderberry into your wellness routine may help support your immune system and provide relief from respiratory symptoms. However, it is important to note that elderberry is not a substitute for medical treatment, and it is always recommended to seek advice from a healthcare professional for proper diagnosis and guidance.

As we continue exploring herbal remedies, we will uncover more natural allies in the fight against the common cold. Nature's pharmacy offers a wide array of options to

enhance your well-being and strengthen your body's defenses.
[End of Section 3]

Section 4: Peppermint - Soothing Congestion and Cough

Peppermint, with its invigorating aroma and cooling properties, is a herb renowned for its ability to provide relief from respiratory symptoms, including congestion and cough. In this section, we will explore how peppermint can help soothe these discomforts associated with the common cold.

1. **Decongestant Properties**: Peppermint contains menthol, a compound known for its decongestant properties. Menthol helps to relax and open up the airways, providing relief from nasal congestion and promoting easier breathing. Inhaling the vapors of peppermint can offer a refreshing sensation and help clear the sinuses.

2. **Soothing Cough**: Peppermint's antitussive (cough-suppressing) properties can help alleviate coughs associated with the common cold. Its soothing effect on the throat can provide relief from irritation and reduce the urge to cough. Peppermint is often used in cough drops, lozenges, and teas for its cough-calming benefits.

3. **Inhalation and Steam Therapy**: Inhaling peppermint steam can be especially beneficial for respiratory relief. Add a few drops of peppermint essential oil to a bowl of hot water, place a towel over your head, and inhale the steam for a few minutes. The soothing and aromatic vapors of

peppermint can help ease congestion, unclog the sinuses, and provide temporary relief from coughing.

4. **Peppermint Tea**: Drinking peppermint tea can also provide comfort and relief from cold symptoms. Brew a cup of peppermint tea by steeping dried peppermint leaves in hot water. The warm liquid, combined with the aromatic properties of peppermint, can help soothe the throat, calm coughing, and provide a sense of relief.

5. **Topical Application**: Applying peppermint-infused balms or ointments to the chest, back, or throat can provide a cooling sensation and help alleviate congestion and cough. Gently massaging these preparations onto the skin can promote better blood circulation and provide localized relief.

6. **Safety Considerations**: While peppermint is generally safe for most individuals when used appropriately, some people may experience allergic reactions or sensitivities to peppermint. It is always recommended to perform a patch test before using any topical preparations and consult with a healthcare professional if you have any concerns or underlying health conditions.

Peppermint offers a natural and soothing approach to managing congestion and cough associated with the common cold. However, it is important to remember that peppermint remedies are meant to provide temporary relief and should not replace medical advice or treatment.

As we explore the realm of herbal remedies, we will uncover more natural allies that can support your well-being and aid in the fight against the common cold. Embrace the power of peppermint and nature's bountiful offerings to find comfort and relief during your journey to wellness. [End of Section 4]

Chapter 4

Healing Soups and Broths

Section 1: Chicken Soup - Traditional Cold Fighter

Chicken soup has long been hailed as a comforting and nourishing remedy for the common cold. In this section, we will explore the benefits of chicken soup and how it can help alleviate cold symptoms and support the healing process.

1. **Soothing and Hydrating**: Chicken soup provides comfort and hydration, which are crucial during illness. The warm broth helps soothe a sore throat, while the liquid content helps keep you hydrated. Staying hydrated is essential for thinning mucus, supporting respiratory health, and preventing dehydration.

2. **Nutrient-Rich Ingredients**: Chicken soup is often prepared with various nutritious ingredients, such as chicken, vegetables, herbs, and spices. These ingredients contribute to the soup's nutrient content,

providing essential vitamins, minerals, and antioxidants that support overall health and immune function.

3. **Anti-Inflammatory Properties**: Chicken soup may have anti-inflammatory effects due to its ingredients, such as onions, garlic, and herbs like thyme or rosemary. These ingredients contain compounds that can help reduce inflammation in the respiratory tract, alleviating congestion and discomfort associated with the common cold.

4. **Support for Respiratory Health**: The steam from a hot bowl of chicken soup can help moisten and soothe the nasal passages, providing temporary relief from congestion and making it easier to breathe. Inhaling the aromas of the soup may also offer a sense of comfort and relaxation.

5. **Boosting Immune Function**: Chicken soup contains nutrients and compounds that can support immune function. The chicken provides protein, which is essential for immune cell production and repair. The vegetables in the soup offer vitamins and antioxidants that aid in maintaining a strong immune system.

6. **Psychological Comfort**: Beyond its physical benefits, chicken soup provides psychological comfort during times of illness. Its warm and familiar aroma, coupled with the act of savoring a bowl of homemade soup, can provide a sense of nurturing and well-being, promoting a positive mindset during recovery.

7. **Homemade Preparation**: While store-bought chicken soup can offer convenience, homemade chicken soup allows you to control the ingredients and customize the flavors according to your preferences. Homemade soups often contain higher

amounts of nutrients and fewer additives compared to packaged varieties.
Remember, chicken soup is not a cure for the common cold, but it can be a valuable addition to your self-care routine. It provides hydration, essential nutrients, and soothing properties that can help ease symptoms and provide comfort during the recovery process.

In the upcoming sections, we will explore additional healing soups and broths that offer nourishment and relief from the common cold. Embrace the comfort and therapeutic benefits of homemade soups as a natural remedy in your journey to wellness.
[End of Section 1]

Section 2: Vegetable Broth - A Comforting Remedy

Vegetable broth, rich in nutrients and flavors, offers a comforting and nourishing alternative for those seeking a vegetarian or vegan option to alleviate cold symptoms. In this section, we will explore the benefits of vegetable broth and how it can provide relief during the common cold.

1. **Nutrient-Packed**: Vegetable broth is packed with an array of nutrients from a variety of vegetables, herbs, and spices. It provides vitamins, minerals, antioxidants, and phytochemicals that support immune function and overall health.
2. **Hydration and Warmth**: Similar to chicken soup, vegetable broth offers hydration and warmth, which are essential during illness. Staying hydrated helps thin mucus, ease congestion, and maintain proper

bodily functions. The warm broth can soothe a sore throat and provide comfort.

3. **Immune-Boosting Ingredients**: Vegetable broth often includes immune-boosting ingredients such as onions, garlic, ginger, turmeric, and mushrooms. These ingredients contain compounds known for their antimicrobial, anti-inflammatory, and antioxidant properties, which can aid in strengthening the immune system.

4. **Respiratory Support**: The steam from a bowl of hot vegetable broth can help moisten the respiratory passages, providing temporary relief from nasal congestion and making breathing more comfortable. Inhaling the aroma of the broth can also have a calming and soothing effect.

5. **Digestive Ease**: During a cold, digestion may be affected. Vegetable broth, with its light and easily digestible nature, provides essential nutrients without putting excess strain on the digestive system. It can be a gentle source of nourishment when appetite is diminished.

6. **Customizable and Versatile**: One of the benefits of vegetable broth is its versatility and customizability. You can tailor the ingredients to suit your taste preferences and dietary needs. Experiment with a variety of vegetables, herbs, and spices to create a flavorful and nutrient-dense broth that resonates with your palate.

7. **Culinary Base**: Vegetable broth serves as a culinary base for other dishes, such as soups, stews, and sauces. By incorporating vegetable broth into your cooking, you can infuse meals with added nutrition and flavor while still enjoying the benefits of its immune-supporting properties.

When preparing vegetable broth, consider using a variety of vegetables like carrots, celery, onions, leeks, kale, and herbs like thyme or parsley. Simmering the ingredients in water for an extended period allows the flavors and nutrients to meld together.

While vegetable broth offers nourishment and comfort, it is important to note that it is not a cure for the common cold. It should be complemented with rest, hydration, and other supportive measures.

In the following sections, we will explore more healing soups and broths, providing you with a repertoire of options to soothe your cold symptoms and support your journey to recovery. Embrace the nourishing power of vegetable broth as a comforting remedy in your pursuit of wellness.
[End of Section 2]

Section 3: Bone Broth - Nutrient-Rich Elixir for Colds

Bone broth, a flavorful liquid made by simmering bones and connective tissues, is a nutrient-rich elixir that has been used for centuries to support health and well-being. In this section, we will explore the benefits of bone broth and its potential as a soothing remedy during the common cold.

1. **Nutrient Density**: Bone broth is rich in essential nutrients, including minerals like calcium, magnesium, and phosphorus, as well as amino acids, collagen, gelatin, and other compounds. These nutrients provide a nourishing boost to support overall health and aid in the healing process.

2. **Immune-Boosting Properties**: Bone broth contains immune-boosting compounds, such as glutamine and arginine, that support immune function. It also contains collagen, which has been linked to gut health and enhanced immune response. A strong immune system is vital for fighting off infections, including the common cold.

3. **Respiratory Comfort**: The steam from a hot cup of bone broth can help soothe the respiratory passages, providing temporary relief from nasal congestion, coughing, and throat irritation. Inhaling the warm vapors can offer a comforting effect, helping to clear the airways and ease breathing.

4. **Gut Health Support**: The gelatin and collagen present in bone broth are beneficial for gut health. A healthy gut is closely linked to a strong immune system. Consuming bone broth can help support the integrity of the gut lining, improve digestion, and aid in nutrient absorption, all of which contribute to overall well-being.

5. **Hydration and Warmth**: Staying hydrated is crucial during illness, and bone broth provides a hydrating option. The warm liquid can help soothe a sore throat, provide comfort, and maintain proper hydration levels. Adequate hydration supports the thinning of mucus, making it easier to clear congestion.

6. **Homemade Preparation**: While commercially available bone broths are an option, preparing bone broth at home allows you to have control over the ingredients and quality. You can use a variety of bones, such as chicken, beef, or fish, and simmer them with aromatic vegetables, herbs, and spices to create a flavorful and nutrient-dense broth.

7. **Versatility**: Bone broth serves as a versatile base for other soups, stews, and dishes. It can be enjoyed on its own or used as a flavorful addition to various recipes, providing both taste and nutritional benefits.

It is important to note that some individuals, such as those with certain health conditions or dietary restrictions, may need to consult with a healthcare professional or registered dietitian before incorporating bone broth into their routine. While bone broth can be a nourishing addition to your cold-fighting arsenal, it is not a substitute for medical treatment or professional advice. It should be used in conjunction with other supportive measures, such as rest, hydration, and appropriate medical care when needed.

As we continue our exploration of healing soups and broths, we will uncover more options to soothe your cold symptoms and promote overall well-being. Embrace the healing potential of bone broth as a nutrient-rich elixir during your journey to recovery.

[End of Section 3]

Chapter 5

Hot Drinks and Teas

Section 1: Lemon and Honey Tea - Soothing Sore Throat

Lemon and honey tea is a comforting and soothing beverage that has been used for generations to provide relief from a sore throat and support the healing process. In this section, we will explore the benefits of lemon and honey tea and how it can help alleviate discomfort during the common cold.

1. **Soothing and Hydrating**: Lemon and honey tea offers soothing properties that can help alleviate the pain and irritation of a sore throat. The warmth of the tea provides comfort, while the lemon and honey provide a soothing coating effect, reducing discomfort and inflammation. Additionally, the liquid content helps keep you hydrated, which is crucial for thinning mucus and supporting overall well-being.

2. **Vitamin C Boost**: Lemons are a rich source of vitamin C, a powerful antioxidant that supports immune function. Adding lemon juice to your tea can provide a vitamin C boost, which may help

strengthen your immune system and aid in fighting off the common cold.

3. **Antibacterial and Antimicrobial Properties**: Both lemon and honey possess antibacterial and antimicrobial properties. Lemon contains compounds that can help inhibit the growth of bacteria, while honey has been used for centuries for its antimicrobial properties. These properties may help combat the bacteria that contribute to a sore throat.

4. **Cough Relief**: Honey has long been recognized for its natural cough-suppressing properties. It forms a soothing layer in the throat, reducing irritation and helping to calm coughing. Incorporating honey into your lemon tea can provide temporary relief from coughing and promote a more comfortable throat.

5. **Flavorful and Aromatic**: Lemon and honey tea offers a delightful flavor and aroma that can uplift your spirits during illness. The tanginess of lemon and the sweetness of honey create a balanced and enjoyable taste experience, making the tea a pleasant and comforting beverage.

6. **Simple Preparation**: Preparing lemon and honey tea is a straightforward process. Squeeze the juice of fresh lemon into a cup, add a spoonful of honey, and pour hot water over the mixture. Stir well until the honey is dissolved. Adjust the lemon and honey amounts to suit your taste preferences.

Remember, while lemon and honey tea can provide temporary relief from a sore throat and offer soothing benefits, it is not a substitute for medical treatment or professional advice. It should be used in conjunction with other appropriate measures to support your recovery.

In the subsequent sections, we will explore more hot drinks and teas that offer comfort and relief during the common

cold. Embrace the warmth and healing properties of these beverages as you embark on your journey to wellness.
[End of Section 1]

Section 2: Turmeric Milk - Anti-inflammatory Elixir

Turmeric milk, also known as golden milk, is a popular beverage cherished for its anti-inflammatory properties and potential to soothe cold symptoms. In this section, we will explore the benefits of turmeric milk and how it can serve as an anti-inflammatory elixir during the common cold.

1. **Anti-inflammatory Effects**: Turmeric contains curcumin, a bioactive compound known for its potent anti-inflammatory properties. Consuming turmeric milk can help reduce inflammation in the body, alleviating symptoms such as nasal congestion, sore throat, and cough associated with the common cold.

2. **Immune Support**: Curcumin in turmeric also exhibits immune-modulating effects. By supporting immune function, turmeric milk can help bolster your body's natural defense mechanisms, making it more resilient against infections, including the common cold.

3. **Soothing and Comforting**: Turmeric milk offers a soothing and comforting experience. The warm milk combined with the earthy flavors of turmeric, cinnamon, and other spices creates a delightful beverage that promotes relaxation and a sense of well-being during times of illness.

4. **Respiratory Relief**: Turmeric milk may help ease respiratory symptoms associated with the common

cold. The anti-inflammatory properties of turmeric, along with the warming effects of the drink, can help soothe irritated airways, reduce congestion, and promote easier breathing.

5. **Antioxidant Support**: Turmeric is rich in antioxidants, which help protect against cellular damage caused by oxidative stress. Antioxidants aid in strengthening the immune system and reducing inflammation, further supporting the body's ability to fight off infections.

6. **Nutritional Benefits**: Turmeric milk is often prepared with milk or plant-based milk alternatives, such as almond or coconut milk. These milk options offer additional nutrients like protein, calcium, and vitamins, which contribute to overall nutrition and support immune function.

7. **Customizable Preparation**: Turmeric milk can be customized to suit individual preferences. You can adjust the amount of turmeric, spices, and sweeteners according to your taste. Including other beneficial ingredients like ginger, cinnamon, or honey can further enhance the flavor and health benefits of the beverage.

It's important to note that curcumin, the active compound in turmeric, may have limited absorption in the body. Combining turmeric with black pepper or consuming it with a source of fat (such as milk) can improve its absorption.

While turmeric milk offers potential health benefits, it should not replace medical treatment or professional advice. It is recommended to consult with a healthcare professional before incorporating turmeric milk into your routine, especially if you have specific health conditions or are taking medications.

As we explore more hot drinks and teas, we will uncover additional soothing options to provide comfort and relief during the common cold. Embrace the anti-inflammatory properties of turmeric milk as an elixir for wellness on your journey to recovery.
[End of Section 2]

Section 3: Chamomile Tea - Calming Respiratory Remedy

Chamomile tea, known for its gentle and soothing qualities, serves as a calming respiratory remedy during the common cold. In this section, we will explore the benefits of chamomile tea and how it can help alleviate respiratory discomfort associated with cold symptoms.

1. **Relaxing and Calming**: Chamomile tea is revered for its calming properties, which can provide a sense of relaxation during illness. The gentle aroma and warmth of the tea can help ease tension and promote a state of calmness, aiding in restful sleep and overall well-being.
2. **Throat Soothing**: Chamomile tea has a soothing effect on the throat, making it beneficial for alleviating soreness, irritation, and coughing. The anti-inflammatory properties of chamomile can help reduce inflammation and promote comfort in the respiratory tract.
3. **Respiratory Support**: Drinking chamomile tea may provide respiratory support during the common cold. The warm tea can help loosen mucus and relieve congestion, making it easier to breathe. It can also help calm irritated airways, reducing coughing and promoting a sense of ease.

4. **Immune-Boosting Properties**: Chamomile contains compounds with potential immune-boosting properties, such as flavonoids and antioxidants. While further research is needed, these compounds may support immune function, helping the body fight off infections and recover from illnesses like the common cold.

5. **Relaxation and Sleep Aid**: Restful sleep is crucial for the body's healing process. Chamomile tea's calming properties can promote relaxation and improve sleep quality, allowing the body to recharge and strengthen its defenses against the cold. Enjoying a cup of chamomile tea before bedtime can facilitate a peaceful night's sleep.

6. **Digestive Comfort**: Chamomile tea is known to aid in digestion and soothe the digestive system. During a cold, digestive discomfort may occur due to factors like mucus drainage or changes in appetite. Drinking chamomile tea can help ease digestive symptoms, such as bloating or indigestion, providing additional relief during illness.

7. **Customizable Preparation**: Chamomile tea is readily available in tea bags or loose-leaf form, allowing you to adjust the strength and flavor according to your preferences. You can enhance the tea's benefits by adding a touch of honey or lemon for added soothing and immune-supporting properties.

While chamomile tea offers potential benefits, it should not replace medical treatment or professional advice. It is advisable to consult with a healthcare professional if you have specific health conditions, allergies, or concerns.

As we continue exploring hot drinks and teas, we will uncover more options to provide comfort and relief during the common cold. Embrace the calming and respiratory

support of chamomile tea as a gentle remedy on your path
to wellness.
[End of Section 3]

Chapter 6

Steam and Inhalation Therapy

Section 1: Eucalyptus Steam-Clearing Nasal Passages

Steam and inhalation therapy can be beneficial in relieving congestion and clearing nasal passages during the common cold. In this section, we will explore the use of eucalyptus steam as an effective method for promoting respiratory comfort.

1. **Eucalyptus Benefits**: Eucalyptus is known for its decongestant properties, making it a popular choice for steam inhalation therapy. The aromatic compounds found in eucalyptus oil, such as eucalyptol, can help reduce nasal congestion, open up the airways, and promote easier breathing.

2. **Steam's Moisturizing Effect**: Steam inhalation provides moist heat that helps hydrate and soothe irritated respiratory passages. The warm, moist air can help thin mucus, making it easier to expel and

reducing nasal congestion. It can also alleviate dryness and irritation in the nose and throat.

3. **Sinus and Nasal Relief**: Eucalyptus steam can specifically target sinus and nasal discomfort. The inhalation of eucalyptus-infused steam can help loosen mucus and relieve pressure in the sinuses, providing relief from congestion, sinus headaches, and sinus-related pain.

4. **Antimicrobial Properties**: Eucalyptus possesses natural antimicrobial properties, which may help combat bacteria and viruses that contribute to respiratory infections. Inhaling eucalyptus steam can create an inhospitable environment for these pathogens, aiding in the body's defense against the common cold.

5. **Preparation and Safety**: To create eucalyptus steam, add a few drops of eucalyptus essential oil to a bowl of hot water. Position your face over the bowl, covering your head with a towel to trap the steam, and inhale deeply. Be cautious not to get too close to the hot water to prevent burns. Start with short sessions and gradually increase duration as tolerated.

6. **Cautionary Notes**: Eucalyptus oil should be used with care, as it is potent and can be irritating to some individuals, especially those with sensitive skin or respiratory conditions. If you have any concerns or are uncertain about using eucalyptus oil, consult with a healthcare professional or aromatherapist before proceeding.

7. **Additional Considerations**: Inhaling eucalyptus steam can provide temporary relief from congestion and promote respiratory comfort. However, it is important to remember that steam inhalation is not a substitute for medical treatment or professional

advice. It should be used in conjunction with other appropriate measures to support your recovery.

As we delve further into steam and inhalation therapy, we will explore additional methods to help alleviate respiratory symptoms during the common cold. Embrace the power of eucalyptus steam as a natural aid in clearing your nasal passages and promoting a sense of respiratory relief.
[End of Section 1]

Section 2: Saltwater Gargle - Relieving Sore Throat

A saltwater gargle is a simple yet effective home remedy for relieving a sore throat, a common symptom of the common cold. In this section, we will explore the benefits of saltwater gargle and how it can provide relief during your recovery.

1. **Soothing and Hydrating**: A saltwater gargle can help soothe a sore throat by reducing inflammation and providing temporary relief. The warm saltwater can also help hydrate the throat, alleviating dryness and discomfort associated with a sore throat.

2. **Salt's Antiseptic Properties**: Salt possesses antiseptic properties, which can help inhibit the growth of bacteria in the throat. Gargling with saltwater can create an environment that is less conducive to bacterial growth, potentially reducing the risk of infection and promoting a faster recovery.

3. **Mucus and Irritant Removal**: Gargling with saltwater can help loosen and remove mucus, phlegm, and irritants that may be lingering in the throat. This action can provide relief from

congestion and reduce the frequency of coughing caused by postnasal drip.

4. **Reducing Swelling**: Saltwater gargling can help reduce swelling in the throat, minimizing discomfort and easing swallowing difficulties. By reducing inflammation, it can promote a more comfortable throat, allowing you to stay hydrated and nourished during the healing process.

5. **Simple Preparation**: To prepare a saltwater gargle, dissolve half a teaspoon of salt in warm water. Stir until the salt is completely dissolved. Take a sip of the mixture, tilt your head back, and gargle for 15-30 seconds before spitting it out. Repeat the process as needed, ensuring not to swallow the solution.

6. **Frequency and Safety**: Gargling with saltwater can be done multiple times a day, depending on the severity of your symptoms. However, it's important not to swallow the solution, as it can dehydrate your body. If you have specific health conditions or concerns, consult with a healthcare professional before using a saltwater gargle.

7. **Supplemental Tips**: To enhance the effects of a saltwater gargle, you can consider adding additional ingredients such as a small amount of baking soda or a few drops of honey for added soothing properties. These additions can help further relieve soreness and provide comfort.

While a saltwater gargle can provide temporary relief from a sore throat, it should not replace medical treatment or professional advice. It is important to seek appropriate medical care and follow the guidance of healthcare professionals for a comprehensive approach to your recovery.

As we explore additional remedies, we will uncover more ways to alleviate symptoms and promote well-being during the common cold. Embrace the simplicity and effectiveness of a saltwater gargle as a soothing remedy for your sore throat on your path to healing.
[End of Section 2]

Section 3: Inhalation with Essential Oils - Easing Congestion

Inhalation therapy with essential oils can be a valuable tool for easing congestion during the common cold. In this section, we will explore how inhaling essential oils can help clear nasal passages and promote respiratory comfort.

1. **Decongestant Effects**: Essential oils, such as eucalyptus, peppermint, and tea tree oil, possess natural decongestant properties. Inhaling these oils can help reduce nasal congestion, open up the airways, and alleviate breathing difficulties caused by a cold.

2. **Anti-inflammatory Properties**: Certain essential oils, like lavender, chamomile, and frankincense, have anti-inflammatory properties that can help reduce inflammation in the respiratory tract. By inhaling these oils, you may experience relief from swollen nasal passages and a decreased sensation of congestion.

3. **Respiratory Support**: Inhalation therapy with essential oils can provide respiratory support by promoting clearer breathing and helping to thin and expel mucus. The aromatic compounds of the oils

can help break up congestion, making it easier to clear the airways and breathe more comfortably.

4. **Steam Inhalation**: One method of inhaling essential oils is through steam inhalation. Add a few drops of your chosen essential oil to a bowl of hot water, place a towel over your head to create a tent, and inhale the aromatic steam deeply. This allows the essential oil vapors to reach your respiratory system, providing relief from congestion.

5. **Diffusion**: Another way to inhale essential oils is through the use of a diffuser. Diffusers disperse the oils into the air, allowing you to breathe in the beneficial properties of the oils over an extended period. This method can be especially helpful in creating a soothing and healing environment in your home.

6. **Dilution and Safety**: It is important to dilute essential oils properly before inhalation or use. Essential oils are highly concentrated and can be irritating if used undiluted. Follow recommended dilution ratios and safety guidelines provided by reputable sources or consult with an aromatherapist or healthcare professional for personalized guidance.

7. **Personal Preferences**: Essential oils vary in aroma and properties, so it's essential to choose oils that resonate with you and suit your individual needs. Experiment with different oils and find the scents and combinations that provide the most relief and comfort for your congestion.

While inhalation therapy with essential oils can provide temporary relief from congestion, it should not replace medical treatment or professional advice. If you have specific health conditions, allergies, or concerns, it is advisable to consult with a healthcare professional or aromatherapist before using essential oils.

As we explore additional remedies, we will uncover more natural ways to alleviate congestion and promote respiratory well-being during the common cold. Embrace the power of essential oils and inhalation therapy as a comforting remedy on your journey to clearer breathing and improved comfort.

Chapter 7

Rest and Sleep

Section 1: Importance of Rest in Recovery

Rest and sleep play a crucial role in the recovery process during the common cold. In this section, we will explore the importance of rest and how it aids in your body's healing journey.

1. **Healing and Repair**: Rest provides an opportunity for your body to focus its energy on healing and repairing itself. When you rest, your immune system can work more efficiently to fight off the viral infection that causes the common cold. It allows your body's resources to be directed towards recovery and restoring balance.

2. **Energy Conservation**: When you rest, you conserve energy that can be utilized by your immune system to combat the cold virus. By conserving energy, you optimize your body's ability to function and heal. This is especially important as

the common cold can often leave you feeling fatigued and drained.

3. **Reduced Stress**: Rest can help reduce stress levels, allowing your body to better manage the immune response and inflammatory processes associated with the cold. Chronic stress can negatively impact your immune system, making it more difficult for your body to fight off infections. Rest serves as a natural stress reducer, supporting a healthier immune system response.

4. **Symptom Management**: Rest can alleviate symptoms and discomfort associated with the common cold. Taking the time to rest gives your body the chance to recover and provides relief from symptoms such as fatigue, body aches, headache, and congestion. It allows your body to replenish energy reserves and regain strength.

5. **Sleep Quality**: Quality sleep is vital for immune function and overall well-being. During sleep, your body produces and releases essential hormones that regulate immune responses and repair cellular damage. Adequate sleep strengthens your immune system and supports your body's ability to fight off infections effectively.

6. **Promoting Recovery**: Rest and sleep help shorten the duration of the common cold. By giving your body the rest it needs, you allow it to efficiently utilize its resources to combat the virus and expedite the recovery process. Getting sufficient rest can help you bounce back more quickly and regain your optimal health.

7. **Self-Care and Wellness**: Rest is an act of self-care and an investment in your overall wellness. Prioritizing rest during the common cold allows you to listen to your body's needs, honor its limits, and

provide it with the nurturing environment it requires
to heal. Rest is an essential component of
maintaining a healthy lifestyle.
Remember to listen to your body and give yourself
permission to rest when you need it during the common
cold. It is a valuable and necessary part of your recovery
journey. While rest is beneficial, it is also important to seek
medical attention if your symptoms worsen or persist.

As we continue to explore ways to support your well-being
during the common cold, we will uncover additional
strategies to optimize rest and sleep. Embrace the power of
rest as a foundational pillar in your path to recovery and
enhanced overall wellness.
[End of Section 1]

Section 2: Tips for Improving Sleep During a Cold

Getting quality sleep is crucial for supporting your
immune system and aiding in the recovery process during
a cold. In this section, we will explore practical tips to help
improve sleep despite the discomfort of cold symptoms.

1. **Elevate your head**: If congestion is making it
   difficult to breathe while lying flat, try propping up
   your head with an extra pillow or using a wedge
   pillow to elevate your upper body. This can help
   alleviate nasal congestion and promote easier
   breathing, allowing for better sleep.

2. **Create a comfortable sleep environment**: Ensure
   your sleep environment is conducive to rest by
   keeping the room cool, dark, and quiet. Use
   earplugs, a sleep mask, or a white noise machine if

needed to minimize disruptions and create a soothing atmosphere.

3. **Stay hydrated**: Drink plenty of fluids throughout the day to stay hydrated, but be mindful of not consuming excessive fluids close to bedtime to avoid frequent nighttime bathroom trips. Maintaining proper hydration can help prevent dryness in the throat and nasal passages, promoting more comfortable sleep.

4. **Nasal irrigation**: Consider using a saline nasal spray or a neti pot to rinse your nasal passages before bed. This can help clear congestion and reduce nasal swelling, making it easier to breathe and promoting better sleep.

5. **Steam inhalation**: Engage in steam inhalation therapy before bedtime using essential oils or plain hot water. Inhaling the warm steam can help loosen mucus, alleviate congestion, and provide respiratory relief, facilitating better sleep.

6. **Warm showers or baths**: Taking a warm shower or bath before bed can help relax your body and relieve muscle tension. The warm water can also provide soothing relief for sore throat and nasal congestion, promoting a more peaceful sleep.

7. **Herbal teas**: Sip on warm herbal teas, such as chamomile or peppermint tea, before bedtime. These teas can have calming properties, promoting relaxation and aiding in better sleep. Be mindful of choosing caffeine-free options to avoid sleep disruptions.

8. **Over-the-counter remedies**: Consider using over-the-counter cold remedies that provide relief specifically for nighttime symptoms. These may include decongestants, cough suppressants, or antihistamines designed to alleviate symptoms and

promote better sleep during a cold. Consult with a pharmacist or healthcare professional to find the right option for you.

9. **Practice relaxation techniques**: Engage in relaxation techniques before bed, such as deep breathing exercises, meditation, or gentle stretching. These practices can help calm your mind and relax your body, preparing you for a restful night's sleep.

10. **Follow a consistent sleep schedule**: Maintain a regular sleep schedule by going to bed and waking up at consistent times. Establishing a routine can help regulate your body's internal clock and improve sleep quality, even during a cold.

Remember, while these tips can enhance sleep quality during a cold, it is important to seek appropriate medical care and follow the guidance of healthcare professionals for a comprehensive approach to your recovery.

As we continue to explore ways to support your well-being during the common cold, we will uncover additional strategies to improve sleep and enhance your overall restorative experience. Embrace these tips as valuable tools to optimize your sleep and aid in your journey to wellness. [End of Section 2]

Section 3: Creating a Conducive Sleep Environment

Creating a sleep-friendly environment is essential for promoting restful sleep, especially during a cold when quality sleep is crucial for recovery. In this section, we will explore tips for setting up a conducive sleep environment to maximize your sleep comfort and support healing.

1. **Comfortable Bed and Bedding**: Invest in a comfortable mattress and pillows that provide adequate support for your body. Choose bedding materials that are soft, breathable, and appropriate for the climate. Ensuring physical comfort is essential for achieving a restful sleep environment.

2. **Temperature Control**: Maintain a cool and comfortable room temperature for sleep, usually between 60-67°F (15-19°C). Adjust the thermostat or use a fan to create a pleasant sleep environment. Experiment with different temperature settings to find what works best for your comfort.

3. **Darkness and Light**: Create a dark sleep environment by using blackout curtains or an eye mask to block out external light sources. This can promote melatonin production, the hormone that regulates sleep, and help you fall asleep faster. Consider using a nightlight or dimming the lights if you need some illumination during the night.

4. **Noise Reduction**: Minimize noise disruptions by using earplugs, white noise machines, or soothing sounds like nature sounds or calming music. These can mask or reduce distracting noises and create a peaceful sleep atmosphere.

5. **Clutter-Free Space**: Maintain a clean and clutter-free bedroom to create a calming atmosphere conducive to relaxation. A tidy space promotes a sense of calm and can help alleviate stress or anxiety that may interfere with sleep.

6. **Scent and Aromatherapy**: Consider incorporating relaxing scents into your sleep environment. Lavender, chamomile, or other calming essential oils or sprays can create a soothing atmosphere and aid in relaxation before bedtime. Use them

sparingly and follow proper dilution and safety guidelines.

7. **Limit Electronics**: Keep electronic devices, such as smartphones, tablets, and televisions, out of the bedroom or establish strict usage guidelines. The blue light emitted by screens can disrupt sleep patterns and interfere with the production of melatonin. Opt for relaxing activities like reading a book or listening to calming music instead.

8. **Establish a Bedtime Routine**: Create a relaxing bedtime routine to signal to your body that it's time to unwind and prepare for sleep. Engage in activities like reading, gentle stretching, taking a warm bath, or practicing relaxation techniques. Consistency in your routine can help signal your body to wind down and prepare for rest.

9. **Proper Ventilation**: Ensure good airflow in your sleep environment by opening windows or using a fan. Fresh air and proper ventilation can help maintain a comfortable sleep environment and promote a sense of well-being.

10. **Personalized Comfort**: Consider personal preferences to create a sleep environment that suits your individual needs. Experiment with different elements, such as room temperature, bedding materials, scents, and ambient sounds, to find what promotes optimal sleep and relaxation for you.

By implementing these tips, you can create a sleep environment that supports restful sleep, allowing your body to heal and recover more effectively during a cold.

As we continue to explore ways to enhance your well-being during the common cold, we will uncover additional strategies to improve sleep and promote a nurturing sleep environment. Embrace these tips as tools to optimize your sleep and support your journey to wellness.

Chapter 8

Nasal Irrigation and Saline Rinse

Section 1: Neti Pot - Clearing Nasal Congestion

Nasal irrigation, including the use of a neti pot, is a natural and effective method for clearing nasal congestion during the common cold. In this section, we will explore the benefits of using a neti pot and how it can provide relief from congestion.

1. **Sinus Clearing**: A neti pot is a small container used to flush out the nasal passages with a saline solution. By gently pouring the saline solution through one nostril and letting it flow out through the other, the neti pot helps clear mucus, allergens, and irritants from the sinuses. This can alleviate nasal congestion and promote easier breathing.

2. **Moisturizing Effect**: Nasal irrigation with a neti pot helps hydrate the nasal passages and prevent dryness. Dry nasal passages can contribute to discomfort and irritation during a cold. The saline

solution used in a neti pot provides a gentle moisturizing effect, soothing the nasal tissues and reducing congestion-related discomfort.

3. **Mucus Thinning**: The saline solution used in a neti pot helps thin and loosen mucus, making it easier to expel. This can be particularly beneficial during a cold when excess mucus can contribute to congestion and postnasal drip. By clearing the nasal passages, a neti pot can provide relief from a stuffy nose and improve breathing.

4. **Reduction of Irritants and Allergens**: Nasal irrigation with a neti pot can help remove irritants, allergens, and bacteria that may be present in the nasal passages. Flushing these substances out of the nasal cavities can reduce inflammation and alleviate symptoms such as sneezing, itching, and nasal congestion.

5. **Sinus Pressure Relief**: When the nasal passages are congested, sinus pressure can build up, leading to discomfort and headaches. Using a neti pot can help relieve sinus pressure by clearing the nasal passages and allowing proper drainage, thus reducing pain and congestion in the sinus cavities.

6. **Easy to Use**: Using a neti pot is a relatively simple process. Begin by preparing a saline solution using distilled or sterilized water mixed with a proper amount of salt. Follow the instructions provided with the neti pot for the correct technique. Tilt your head to the side and pour the saline solution into one nostril, allowing it to flow out through the other nostril. Repeat on the other side. Be sure to use only sterile water and follow proper hygiene practices to prevent any risk of infection.

7. **Precautions and Hygiene**: It is important to use only distilled or sterilized water and proper saline

solutions when using a neti pot to prevent the risk of infection. Ensure the neti pot is clean and dry before each use. Follow the instructions carefully and maintain good hygiene practices to avoid any potential complications.

While a neti pot can provide relief from nasal congestion, it should not replace medical treatment or professional advice. If you have specific health conditions, nasal abnormalities, or concerns, consult with a healthcare professional before using a neti pot.

As we continue to explore remedies for nasal congestion during the common cold, we will uncover additional strategies to promote clear breathing and nasal comfort. Embrace the benefits of nasal irrigation and the use of a neti pot as a natural aid in alleviating congestion and promoting overall respiratory well-being.

[End of Section 1]

Section 2: Saline Rinse - Moisturizing Nasal Passages

Saline rinses are a gentle and effective method for moisturizing the nasal passages during the common cold. In this section, we will explore the benefits of saline rinses and how they can provide relief from dryness and discomfort.

1. **Nasal Moisturization**: Saline rinses help moisturize the nasal passages, which can become dry and irritated during a cold. The saline solution, consisting of salt and water, provides a gentle and hydrating effect on the nasal tissues, relieving dryness and reducing discomfort.

2. **Soothing Irritation**: The saline solution used in rinses soothes irritated nasal passages. It helps alleviate symptoms such as itching, burning, or stinging sensations that may arise from dryness and inflammation. The gentle nature of the saline rinse provides relief without causing further irritation.

3. **Loosening Mucus**: Saline rinses can help thin and loosen mucus, making it easier to expel from the nasal passages. This can be particularly helpful during a cold when excess mucus can contribute to congestion and postnasal drip. By promoting mucus clearance, saline rinses aid in maintaining clear and comfortable nasal passages.

4. **Clearing Allergens and Irritants**: Saline rinses effectively flush out allergens, irritants, and bacteria that may be present in the nasal passages. This helps reduce inflammation and remove substances that can trigger allergies or worsen cold symptoms. By clearing the nasal passages, saline rinses contribute to a cleaner and healthier nasal environment.

5. **Enhancing Sinus Health**: Regular use of saline rinses can promote sinus health by maintaining proper nasal hygiene. By keeping the nasal passages moisturized and free from excess mucus and irritants, saline rinses help prevent sinus infections and reduce the risk of sinus-related complications during a cold.

6. **Convenient and Safe**: Saline rinses are readily available in pre-packaged saline solutions or can be prepared at home using sterile water and salt. They are easy to use and generally safe for most individuals. Follow the instructions provided with the saline rinse product or consult with a healthcare professional for proper usage and hygiene practices.

7. **Personalized Approach**: There are different delivery methods for saline rinses, including squeeze bottles, nasal sprays, or neti pots. Experiment with various options to find the method that works best for you and provides optimal comfort and relief.

While saline rinses can provide relief from dry nasal passages, they should not replace medical treatment or professional advice. If you have specific health conditions, nasal abnormalities, or concerns, consult with a healthcare professional before using saline rinses.

As we continue to explore remedies for nasal discomfort during the common cold, we will uncover additional strategies to promote nasal moisture and overall respiratory well-being. Embrace the benefits of saline rinses as a natural and soothing aid in moisturizing your nasal passages and enhancing your comfort during the recovery process.

[End of Section 2]

Chapter 9

Warm Compresses and Chest Rubs

Section 1: Warm Compress - Relieving Sinus Pressure

Warm compresses can be a simple and effective method for relieving sinus pressure and promoting comfort during the common cold. In this section, we will explore the benefits of using a warm compress and how it can provide relief from sinus-related symptoms.

1. **Sinus Pressure Relief**: A warm compress applied to the sinus area can help alleviate sinus pressure and discomfort caused by congestion. The warmth from the compress helps to soothe the tissues, reduce inflammation, and promote sinus drainage, providing relief from sinus-related symptoms.

2. **Promoting Sinus Drainage**: By applying a warm compress, you can encourage the loosening and thinning of mucus in the sinus cavities. This can aid in the natural drainage process, allowing mucus to

flow more freely and relieving congestion and pressure.

3. **Soothing Effect**: The warmth from a compress has a calming and soothing effect on the sinus area. It can help relax the muscles and tissues, reducing tension and promoting overall comfort. This can be particularly beneficial when experiencing sinus headaches or facial pain during a cold.

4. **Easy to Use**: Using a warm compress is simple and convenient. You can create a warm compress by soaking a clean washcloth in warm water and wringing out the excess moisture. Ensure the temperature is comfortably warm but not too hot to avoid burns. Apply the warm compress to the sinus area, such as the forehead or cheeks, and hold it gently for a few minutes at a time.

5. **Steam Inhalation Combination**: For enhanced sinus relief, consider combining a warm compress with steam inhalation therapy. Start by applying a warm compress to the sinus area to promote relaxation and warmth. Then, engage in steam inhalation with essential oils or plain hot water to further alleviate congestion and open up the nasal passages.

6. **Repeat as Needed**: You can use a warm compress multiple times a day or whenever you feel the need for sinus pressure relief. Customize the frequency and duration based on your comfort and symptom severity. Ensure to follow proper hygiene practices and use a clean compress for each application.

7. **Seek Medical Attention**: While a warm compress can provide temporary relief from sinus pressure, it should not replace medical treatment or professional advice. If you experience persistent or severe symptoms, or if your condition worsens, it is

important to seek medical attention for a comprehensive evaluation and appropriate treatment.

As we continue to explore remedies for sinus-related symptoms during the common cold, we will uncover additional strategies to promote comfort and alleviate congestion. Embrace the benefits of a warm compress as a natural aid in relieving sinus pressure and enhancing your overall well-being during the recovery process.

[End of Section 1]

Section 2: Homemade Chest Rubs - Natural Congestion Relief

Homemade chest rubs can provide natural relief from congestion during the common cold. In this section, we will explore the benefits of creating your own chest rub and how it can alleviate congestion and promote respiratory comfort.

1. **Congestion Relief**: Homemade chest rubs are formulated with natural ingredients that can help alleviate congestion and ease breathing difficulties. The combination of these ingredients creates a soothing and aromatic balm that can provide temporary relief from nasal and chest congestion.

2. **Eucalyptus and Peppermint Essential Oils**: Eucalyptus and peppermint essential oils are commonly used in homemade chest rubs due to their decongestant properties. These oils can help open up the airways, clear nasal passages, and relieve congestion. They provide a cooling and refreshing sensation that can provide relief from respiratory discomfort.

3. **Soothing and Calming Effects**: Homemade chest rubs often include ingredients like coconut oil, shea butter, or beeswax, which have moisturizing and soothing properties. These ingredients help to nourish and protect the skin while providing a calming effect on the chest and respiratory area.

4. **Aromatherapy Benefits**: In addition to congestion relief, the aromatic properties of the essential oils used in chest rubs can provide additional benefits. Inhalation of the pleasant scents can help promote relaxation, reduce stress, and enhance overall well-being during the recovery process.

5. **Simple DIY Preparation**: Creating a homemade chest rub is relatively simple. Start with a carrier oil, such as coconut oil or olive oil, and melt it gently over low heat. Add a few drops of eucalyptus and peppermint essential oils and stir well. Pour the mixture into a clean container and allow it to solidify. Adjust the essential oil ratios according to your preference, but use them in moderation to avoid skin sensitivities.

6. **Application Techniques**: To use the chest rub, take a small amount and gently massage it onto the chest, back, and throat area. The warmth from your hands will help melt the balm and facilitate absorption. You can apply the chest rub as needed, typically a few times a day or before bedtime, to alleviate congestion and promote respiratory comfort.

7. **Precautions and Allergies**: It is important to be aware of any potential allergies or sensitivities to the ingredients used in the chest rub. Perform a patch test on a small area of skin before applying it more extensively. If you experience any adverse

reactions, discontinue use and consult with a
healthcare professional.
Remember, while homemade chest rubs can provide
temporary relief from congestion, they should not replace
medical treatment or professional advice. If you have
specific health conditions, allergies, or concerns, consult
with a healthcare professional before using chest rubs.

As we continue to explore remedies for congestion relief
during the common cold, we will uncover additional
natural strategies to promote respiratory well-being.
Embrace the benefits of homemade chest rubs as a natural
and aromatic aid in relieving congestion and enhancing
your comfort during the recovery process.
[End of Section 2]

Chapter 10

Essential Oils for Cold Relief

Section 1: Peppermint Oil - Easing Breathing Difficulties

Peppermint oil is a popular essential oil known for its ability to ease breathing difficulties during the common cold. In this section, we will explore the benefits of peppermint oil and how it can provide relief from respiratory symptoms.

1. **Decongestant Properties**: Peppermint oil acts as a natural decongestant, helping to clear nasal passages and alleviate congestion. The active compound in peppermint oil, menthol, has a cooling and soothing effect on the respiratory system, providing relief from breathing difficulties caused by a cold.

2. **Opening Airways**: The inhalation of peppermint oil vapors can help open up the airways, making it easier to breathe. It can help relax the muscles in the respiratory tract, including the bronchial tubes, and

promote smoother airflow. This can be particularly beneficial for individuals experiencing chest congestion or tightness.

3. **Clearing Mucus**: Peppermint oil's expectorant properties assist in thinning and loosening mucus, making it easier to expel. By reducing the thickness of mucus in the respiratory system, peppermint oil can help alleviate postnasal drip and promote clearer breathing.

4. **Soothing Effect**: Peppermint oil has a soothing and cooling effect on the respiratory tract, providing relief from inflammation and irritation. It can help reduce coughing and calm irritated throat tissues, bringing comfort during bouts of cough and sore throat.

5. **Steam Inhalation**: One effective way to utilize peppermint oil is through steam inhalation. Add a few drops of peppermint oil to a bowl of hot water, position your face over the bowl, cover your head with a towel to trap the steam, and inhale deeply. The inhalation of the peppermint-infused steam can provide instant relief by opening up the airways and soothing respiratory discomfort.

6. **Dilution and Safety**: Peppermint oil is highly concentrated, and it is important to dilute it properly before use. Mix a few drops of peppermint oil with a carrier oil, such as coconut oil or sweet almond oil, before applying it topically or using it for steam inhalation. Follow recommended dilution ratios and safety guidelines to prevent skin sensitivities or adverse reactions.

7. **Personalized Approach**: Individual preferences may vary, and it is important to determine the amount of peppermint oil that works best for you. Start with a lower concentration and adjust

accordingly based on your comfort level and response.

8. **Precautions**: Peppermint oil should be used with caution, as it can be strong and may cause skin sensitivities or allergic reactions in some individuals. Avoid applying peppermint oil near the eyes, on broken or damaged skin, or on infants or young children without proper guidance from a healthcare professional.

While peppermint oil can provide temporary relief from respiratory symptoms, it should not replace medical treatment or professional advice. If you have specific health conditions, allergies, or concerns, consult with a healthcare professional or aromatherapist before using peppermint oil.

As we continue to explore essential oils for cold relief, we will uncover additional strategies to promote respiratory comfort and well-being. Embrace the benefits of peppermint oil as a natural aid in easing breathing difficulties and enhancing your overall respiratory experience during the recovery process.
[End of Section 1]

Section 2: Eucalyptus Oil - Decongestant and Expectorant

Eucalyptus oil is a powerful essential oil known for its decongestant and expectorant properties, making it beneficial for relieving respiratory symptoms during the common cold. In this section, we will explore the benefits of eucalyptus oil and how it can help alleviate congestion and promote respiratory comfort.

1. **Decongestant Effect**: Eucalyptus oil acts as a natural decongestant, helping to clear nasal passages and relieve congestion. It contains a compound called cineole, which has the ability to break up mucus and promote easier breathing by opening up the airways. Inhalation of eucalyptus oil vapors can provide immediate relief from nasal congestion.

2. **Expectorant Properties**: Eucalyptus oil serves as an expectorant, facilitating the loosening and expulsion of mucus from the respiratory tract. It can help thin out sticky mucus, making it easier to cough up and expel. By reducing the thickness of mucus, eucalyptus oil aids in clearing the airways and alleviating respiratory discomfort.

3. **Anti-inflammatory Action**: Eucalyptus oil possesses anti-inflammatory properties that can help reduce inflammation in the respiratory system. It can soothe irritated throat tissues, reduce swelling in the bronchial tubes, and ease coughing and sore throat associated with the common cold.

4. **Steam Inhalation**: Steam inhalation with eucalyptus oil is a popular method for experiencing its benefits. Add a few drops of eucalyptus oil to a bowl of hot water, cover your head with a towel, and inhale the steam deeply. The inhalation of eucalyptus-infused steam can provide immediate relief by clearing the airways, reducing congestion, and promoting easier breathing.

5. **Chest Rubs and Balms**: Eucalyptus oil can be included in homemade chest rubs and balms. When applied topically to the chest and throat area, it can help alleviate congestion and provide soothing relief. Combine a few drops of eucalyptus oil with a carrier oil, such as coconut oil or almond oil, and

gently massage the mixture onto the chest to experience its benefits.

6. **Dilution and Safety**: Eucalyptus oil should be properly diluted before use, as it is highly concentrated. Mix a few drops of eucalyptus oil with a carrier oil or use as directed on the product label. Follow recommended dilution ratios and safety guidelines to avoid skin sensitivities or adverse reactions.

7. **Personalized Approach**: Individual responses to eucalyptus oil may vary. Start with a lower concentration and adjust according to your comfort level and desired effects. Some people find the aroma of eucalyptus oil invigorating, while others may prefer a milder scent. Experiment to find the concentration and usage method that works best for you.

8. **Precautions**: Exercise caution when using eucalyptus oil, as it can be potent and may cause skin sensitivities or allergic reactions in some individuals. Avoid direct contact with eyes, sensitive areas, or broken skin. Consult with a healthcare professional or aromatherapist if you have specific health conditions, allergies, or concerns before using eucalyptus oil.

While eucalyptus oil can provide temporary relief from respiratory symptoms, it should not replace medical treatment or professional advice. If you have underlying health conditions, allergies, or concerns, consult with a healthcare professional or aromatherapist for personalized guidance.

As we continue to explore essential oils for cold relief, we will uncover additional strategies to promote respiratory comfort and enhance your overall well-being. Embrace the benefits of eucalyptus oil as a natural aid in decongestion

and expectoration, supporting your respiratory health during the recovery process.
[End of Section 2]

Section 3: Tea Tree Oil - Fighting Bacterial Infections

Tea tree oil is a versatile essential oil known for its potent antimicrobial properties, making it valuable for fighting bacterial infections during the common cold. In this section, we will explore the benefits of tea tree oil and how it can help combat bacterial infections.

1. **Antimicrobial Activity**: Tea tree oil possesses powerful antimicrobial properties, including antibacterial, antiviral, and antifungal effects. It contains a compound called terpinen-4-ol, which is primarily responsible for its antimicrobial activity. These properties make tea tree oil effective in combating various types of bacteria that may contribute to respiratory infections.

2. **Supporting Immune Function**: Tea tree oil can help support the immune system's response to bacterial infections. By enhancing immune function, it aids in the body's ability to fight off harmful bacteria and promote recovery.

3. **Inhalation Therapy**: Inhaling the vapors of tea tree oil can provide respiratory benefits. Add a few drops of tea tree oil to a bowl of hot water, cover your head with a towel, and inhale the steam deeply. The inhalation of tea tree oil-infused steam can help target bacterial infections in the respiratory tract and provide relief from symptoms such as cough, congestion, and sore throat.

4. **Topical Application**: Tea tree oil can be diluted and applied topically to the chest or throat area to aid in fighting bacterial infections. Mix a few drops of tea tree oil with a carrier oil, such as coconut oil or jojoba oil, and gently massage it onto the skin. This can provide localized antimicrobial effects and alleviate respiratory discomfort.

5. **Natural Disinfectant**: Tea tree oil can be used to create a natural disinfectant spray or solution. Dilute tea tree oil with water in a spray bottle and use it to disinfect surfaces, such as doorknobs, countertops, or other items that may harbor bacteria and contribute to the spread of infections.

6. **Precautions and Safety**: Tea tree oil should always be properly diluted before use, as it can cause skin sensitivities or allergic reactions when used undiluted. Follow recommended dilution ratios and safety guidelines. It is important to note that tea tree oil should not be ingested as it can be toxic. External use only.

7. **Patch Test**: Before applying tea tree oil topically, perform a patch test on a small area of skin to ensure you do not have any adverse reactions. Discontinue use if irritation or sensitivities occur and consult with a healthcare professional.

While tea tree oil can provide antimicrobial benefits, it should not replace medical treatment or professional advice. If you have specific health conditions, allergies, or concerns, consult with a healthcare professional or aromatherapist before using tea tree oil.

As we continue to explore essential oils for combating bacterial infections during the common cold, we will uncover additional strategies to promote respiratory health and support your overall well-being. Embrace the benefits

of tea tree oil as a natural aid in fighting bacterial infections and enhancing your recovery process.
[End of Section 3]

Chapter 11

Soothing Sore Throat Remedies

Section 1: Honey and Warm Water Gargle

When faced with a sore throat, a common and effective natural remedy is a honey and warm water gargle. This soothing combination can help alleviate pain and discomfort. Here's how you can prepare and utilize this remedy:

Ingredients:
- 1 to 2 tablespoons of honey
- 1 cup of warm water

Instructions:
1. Begin by heating the water until it is comfortably warm. Make sure it's not too hot to avoid burning your throat.
2. Measure 1 to 2 tablespoons of honey and add them to the warm water.
3. Stir the mixture thoroughly until the honey is completely dissolved.

4. Take a small sip of the honey and warm water mixture, then tilt your head back slightly.
5. Gargle the solution in your throat for approximately 30 seconds to 1 minute, allowing it to reach the back of your throat.
6. Spit out the mixture into a sink or a container. Avoid swallowing it.
7. Repeat the gargling process with the remaining mixture.
8. You can perform this honey and warm water gargle multiple times a day, especially when your throat feels sore or irritated.

Precautions:

- Do not give honey to children under the age of one year, as it carries a risk of infant botulism. Infant botulism is a rare but serious illness caused by the spores of the bacteria Clostridium botulinum, which can be found in honey. The immature digestive system of infants cannot effectively prevent the growth of these spores, potentially leading to botulism poisoning. It is advised to wait until the child is at least one year old before introducing honey. If you have a known allergy to honey or bee products, it's best to avoid using this remedy.
- Consult a healthcare professional if your sore throat persists, worsens, or is accompanied by severe symptoms.

While a honey and warm water gargle can provide temporary relief for a sore throat, it's important to seek medical advice if your symptoms persist or worsen. A healthcare professional can provide a proper diagnosis and recommend appropriate treatment if necessary.

[End of Section 1]

Section 2: Marshmallow Root Tea

Marshmallow root tea is a traditional herbal remedy known for its soothing properties that can help alleviate sore throat symptoms. Marshmallow root contains mucilage, a substance that forms a protective layer and provides relief to inflamed tissues. Here's how you can prepare and use marshmallow root tea:

Ingredients:
- 1 tablespoon of dried marshmallow root
- 1 cup of boiling water

Instructions:
1. Place the dried marshmallow root in a cup or mug.
2. Pour boiling water over the marshmallow root.
3. Let the mixture steep for about 10 to 15 minutes to allow the beneficial compounds to be extracted.
4. After steeping, strain the tea to remove the marshmallow root.
5. You can add a teaspoon of honey or lemon juice for additional soothing effects or flavor, if desired.
6. Allow the tea to cool down to a comfortable temperature.
7. Take small sips of the marshmallow root tea and allow it to coat your throat as you drink it.
8. Drink this tea 2 to 3 times a day or as needed to soothe your sore throat.

Precautions:
- Marshmallow root tea is generally considered safe for most people. However, if you have any underlying health conditions or are taking medications, it's advisable to consult with a healthcare professional before using marshmallow root tea as a remedy.

- If you experience any adverse reactions or allergies after consuming marshmallow root tea, discontinue its use and seek medical attention.

Please note that herbal remedies, including marshmallow root tea, may provide temporary relief for a sore throat, but they do not replace medical advice or treatment. If your symptoms persist or worsen, it is recommended to consult a healthcare professional for a proper evaluation and guidance.

[End of Section 2]

Section 3: Slippery Elm Lozenges

Slippery elm lozenges are a popular natural remedy for soothing a sore throat. Slippery elm contains a gel-like substance called mucilage that can help coat and protect the throat, reducing irritation and discomfort. Here's how you can use slippery elm lozenges:

Instructions:

1. Purchase slippery elm lozenges from a reputable store or pharmacy. Ensure that the lozenges contain pure slippery elm without any additional additives or ingredients.
2. Take one slippery elm lozenge and place it in your mouth.
3. Allow the lozenge to dissolve slowly in your mouth without chewing or swallowing it immediately. This will enable the slippery elm to come into contact with your throat, providing a soothing effect.
4. Follow the recommended dosage instructions on the packaging of the lozenges. Typically, you can take one lozenge every 2 to 4 hours, or as needed, to alleviate throat discomfort.

5. Make sure to drink water before and after taking the lozenge to stay hydrated and help the lozenge dissolve more easily.
6. Continue using slippery elm lozenges as needed to relieve your sore throat symptoms.

Precautions:

- While slippery elm lozenges are generally safe for most people, it's important to check for any potential allergies or sensitivities to slippery elm or other ingredients present in the lozenges. Discontinue use if you experience any adverse reactions and consult a healthcare professional if needed.
- Keep in mind that slippery elm lozenges are intended for temporary relief of symptoms. If your sore throat persists or worsens, or if you experience other severe symptoms, it's essential to seek medical advice for a proper evaluation and appropriate treatment.

Slippery elm lozenges can provide temporary relief and comfort for a sore throat. However, it's important to note that they are not a substitute for medical treatment, especially if your symptoms are severe or persistent. If in doubt, consult with a healthcare professional for guidance.
[End of Section 3]

Chapter 12

Immune-Boosting Foods

Section 1: Citrus Fruits - Rich in Vitamin C

When it comes to supporting and boosting your immune system, including citrus fruits in your diet can be highly beneficial. Citrus fruits such as oranges, lemons, grapefruits, and limes are renowned for their high vitamin C content. Vitamin C plays a crucial role in supporting immune function and is known for its antioxidant properties. Here's why and how you can incorporate citrus fruits into your diet:

Benefits of Citrus Fruits:

Vitamin C Boost: Citrus fruits are among the best sources of vitamin C, a nutrient that helps stimulate the production of white blood cells, which are key players in the immune response. Vitamin C also promotes the production of antibodies, enhances the activity of natural killer cells, and supports the overall functioning of the immune system.

Ways to Incorporate Citrus Fruits:

1. **Fresh Citrus**: Enjoy citrus fruits in their whole, natural form. Peel and eat oranges, grapefruits, or tangerines as a refreshing snack. Make sure to wash them thoroughly before consumption.
2. **Citrus Juices**: Squeeze fresh citrus fruits to make homemade juices. However, keep in mind that store-bought juices may not have the same nutritional benefits as fresh juices due to processing and added sugars.
3. **Citrus Infused Water**: Add slices of lemon, lime, or orange to your water for a flavorful and hydrating immune-boosting beverage.
4. **Citrus in Salads**: Incorporate citrus fruits into your salads for a burst of tangy flavor. Squeeze some fresh lemon or lime juice as a dressing or add orange segments for sweetness.

Precautions:

- Citrus fruits are generally safe for most people. However, if you have any specific medical conditions or allergies, consult with a healthcare professional before significantly increasing your intake of citrus fruits or taking high-dose vitamin C supplements.
- While vitamin C is beneficial for immune health, it's important to maintain a well-balanced diet with a variety of other nutrients and food groups to support overall wellness.

Including citrus fruits in your diet can be a tasty and effective way to boost your vitamin C intake and support your immune system. Remember to combine them with a balanced diet, regular exercise, and a healthy lifestyle for optimal immune health.

[End of Section 1]

Section 2: Garlic - Natural Antimicrobial Agent

Garlic is a popular ingredient in many culinary dishes and has been valued for its potential health benefits for centuries. One of its notable properties is its natural antimicrobial activity, which can help support the immune system. Here's why garlic is considered an immune-boosting food and how you can incorporate it into your diet:

Benefits of Garlic:

1. **Antimicrobial Properties**: Garlic contains a compound called allicin, which has been shown to exhibit antimicrobial effects. It may help fight against bacteria, viruses, and even certain fungal infections. By incorporating garlic into your diet, you can potentially enhance your body's ability to defend against harmful microorganisms.

Ways to Incorporate Garlic:

1. Fresh Garlic: Use fresh garlic cloves in your cooking to infuse dishes with its distinct flavor and immune-boosting properties. Allow crushed or minced garlic to sit for a few minutes before cooking to activate the allicin compound.

2. Roasted Garlic: Roasting garlic can mellow its flavor and make it a versatile addition to various dishes. Simply wrap a whole bulb of garlic in aluminum foil, drizzle it with olive oil, and bake it until the cloves become soft and golden.

3. Garlic Supplements: Garlic supplements such as garlic extract or aged garlic extract are available in capsule form. However, it's important to consult with a healthcare professional before starting any

dietary supplements, as they may interact with certain medications or have contraindications.

Precautions:

- Garlic is generally safe for most people when consumed in moderate amounts as part of a regular diet. However, excessive consumption of garlic may cause digestive discomfort or interact with certain medications, such as blood thinners. If you have any concerns or underlying health conditions, consult with a healthcare professional before significantly increasing your garlic intake or taking garlic supplements.
- Some people may experience allergies or adverse reactions to garlic. If you notice any symptoms like rash, itching, or difficulty breathing after consuming garlic, discontinue its use and seek medical attention.

Garlic can be a flavorful addition to your meals while potentially providing immune-boosting benefits. However, it's important to remember that it is just one component of a well-rounded diet and healthy lifestyle for supporting overall immune health.

[End of Section 2]

Section 3: Yogurt - Probiotic for Immune Support

Yogurt is a delicious and nutritious food that offers several health benefits, including immune support. Specifically, yogurt is known for its probiotic content, which can help promote a healthy balance of bacteria in the gut and positively impact the immune system. Here's why yogurt is considered an immune-boosting food and how you can incorporate it into your diet:

Benefits of Yogurt:
1. **Probiotics**: Yogurt contains live cultures of beneficial bacteria, known as probiotics, such as Lactobacillus and Bifidobacterium strains. These probiotics help maintain a healthy gut microbiome, which plays a crucial role in supporting the immune system. A balanced gut microbiome can enhance immune response, reduce inflammation, and help defend against harmful pathogens.

Ways to Incorporate Yogurt:
1. **Enjoy It Plain**: Opt for plain, unsweetened yogurt to avoid added sugars. You can enjoy it as is or add fresh fruits, nuts, or seeds for additional flavor and nutrients.
2. **Smoothies**: Blend yogurt with fruits, leafy greens, and a liquid of your choice to create a nutritious and immune-boosting smoothie. Add a dash of honey or a natural sweetener if desired.
3. **Yogurt Parfaits**: Layer yogurt with granola, berries, and a drizzle of honey for a wholesome and satisfying breakfast or snack.
4. **Substitute in Recipes**: You can use yogurt as a substitute for sour cream, mayonnaise, or cream in various recipes to add a creamy texture and probiotic benefits.

Precautions:
- While yogurt is generally safe for most people, individuals with lactose intolerance or dairy allergies should choose lactose-free or non-dairy alternatives. These options, such as almond milk or coconut milk yogurt, often contain probiotics as well.
- Check the label when purchasing yogurt to ensure it contains live and active cultures or specifically mentions the presence of probiotics.

- If you have any specific health concerns or conditions, it's advisable to consult with a healthcare professional before incorporating yogurt or probiotics into your diet.

Yogurt can be a tasty and convenient way to introduce probiotics into your diet, supporting your immune system along with overall gut health. Remember to choose plain varieties without added sugars and maintain a balanced and varied diet for optimal immune support.

[End of Section 3]

Chapter 13

Homeopathic Remedies

Section 1: Oscillococcinum - Reducing Flu-Like Symptoms

Oscillococcinum is a popular homeopathic remedy known for its potential to reduce flu-like symptoms during the common cold. In this section, we will explore the benefits of Oscillococcinum and its role in alleviating flu-like symptoms.

1. **Homeopathic Approach:** Oscillococcinum is based on the principles of homeopathy, which involves using highly diluted substances to stimulate the body's natural healing response. It is prepared from duck liver and heart extracts and is available in the form of small pellets.

2. **Reducing Flu-Like Symptoms:** Oscillococcinum is commonly used for the relief of flu-like symptoms such as body aches, fatigue, chills, and fever. It is believed to stimulate the body's defense mechanisms, helping to reduce the duration and

severity of these symptoms during the common cold.

3. **Easy Administration**: Oscillococcinum is easy to administer. Simply dissolve the recommended pellets under the tongue as directed on the product packaging. It is generally well-tolerated and suitable for adults and children.

4. **Non-Drowsy and Non-Addictive**: One advantage of Oscillococcinum is that it is non-drowsy and non-addictive. It does not cause sedation or dependency, making it suitable for individuals who need to remain alert and carry out daily activities.

5. **Early Intervention**: To obtain the best results, it is recommended to take Oscillococcinum at the onset of flu-like symptoms. Starting treatment early may help in reducing the intensity and duration of symptoms.

6. **Complementary Approach**: Oscillococcinum can be used as a complementary approach alongside conventional medical treatment. It is important to consult with a healthcare professional before using homeopathic remedies to ensure compatibility with other medications or treatments.

7. **Individualized Approach**: Homeopathy recognizes the importance of individualized treatment. While Oscillococcinum is a widely used remedy, the response to homeopathic remedies may vary from person to person. It is recommended to follow the recommended dosage and consult with a qualified homeopath or healthcare professional for personalized guidance.

8. **Precautions**: Although Oscillococcinum is generally considered safe, it is important to follow the recommended dosage and consult with a healthcare professional if you have specific health

conditions, allergies, or concerns. If symptoms persist or worsen, seek medical advice.

While Oscillococcinum may provide relief from flu-like symptoms during the common cold, it should not replace medical treatment or professional advice. It is important to consult with a healthcare professional for a comprehensive evaluation and appropriate treatment.

As we continue to explore homeopathic remedies for the common cold, we will uncover additional strategies to support your well-being and enhance your recovery process. Embrace the benefits of Oscillococcinum as a potential aid in reducing flu-like symptoms and promoting your overall health during the common cold.
[End of Section 1]

Section 2: Allium Cepa - Relieving Watery Eyes and Runny Nose

Allium cepa, derived from the onion plant, is a homeopathic remedy often used to relieve symptoms of watery eyes and runny nose during the common cold. In this section, we will explore the benefits of Allium cepa and its role in alleviating these specific symptoms.

1. **Homeopathic Principle**: Allium cepa is prepared using a highly diluted form of the onion plant, following the principles of homeopathy. This dilution process is believed to enhance its therapeutic properties and reduce any potential side effects.

2. **Watery Eyes Relief**: Allium cepa is commonly used to address symptoms of watery, tearing eyes caused by the common cold. It can help alleviate

excessive tearing and soothe eye irritation, providing relief and improving overall comfort.

3. **Runny Nose Relief**: Another key benefit of Allium cepa is its ability to relieve a runny nose. It is particularly useful when the nasal discharge is profuse and watery, often accompanied by frequent sneezing. Allium cepa helps reduce nasal secretions and congestion, promoting a clearer nasal passage.

4. **Soothing Effect**: Allium cepa has a soothing effect on the mucous membranes. It helps reduce inflammation and irritation in the nasal passages and eyes, providing a comforting sensation and easing discomfort caused by cold-related symptoms.

5. **Individualized Treatment**: Homeopathy recognizes the importance of individualized treatment. While Allium cepa is commonly used for watery eyes and runny nose, the response to homeopathic remedies may vary from person to person. It is recommended to follow the recommended dosage and consult with a qualified homeopath or healthcare professional for personalized guidance.

6. **Easy Administration**: Allium cepa is typically available in the form of small pellets. They can be dissolved under the tongue as directed on the product packaging. It is generally well-tolerated and suitable for adults and children.

7. **Complementary Approach**: Allium cepa can be used as a complementary approach alongside conventional medical treatment. It is important to consult with a healthcare professional before using homeopathic remedies to ensure compatibility with other medications or treatments.

8. **Precautions**: Although Allium cepa is generally considered safe, it is important to follow the

recommended dosage and consult with a healthcare professional if you have specific health conditions, allergies, or concerns. If symptoms persist or worsen, seek medical advice.

While Allium cepa may provide relief from watery eyes and runny nose during the common cold, it should not replace medical treatment or professional advice. It is important to consult with a healthcare professional for a comprehensive evaluation and appropriate treatment.

As we continue to explore homeopathic remedies for the common cold, we will uncover additional strategies to support your well-being and enhance your recovery process. Embrace the benefits of Allium cepa as a potential aid in relieving watery eyes and runny nose, promoting your overall health during the common cold.
[End of Section 2]

Section 3: Nux Vomica - Alleviating Congestion and Headaches

Nux vomica is a homeopathic remedy often used to alleviate congestion and headaches during the common cold. In this section, we will explore the benefits of Nux vomica and its role in providing relief from these specific symptoms.

1. **Homeopathic Principle**: Nux vomica is prepared using a highly diluted form of the Strychnos nux-vomica tree, following the principles of homeopathy. This dilution process enhances its therapeutic properties and reduces the risk of side effects.

2. **Congestion Relief**: Nux vomica is commonly used to address nasal congestion during the common cold. It helps reduce the sensation of blockage and promotes easier breathing by supporting the body's natural response to congestion.

3. **Headache Relief**: Another key benefit of Nux vomica is its potential to alleviate headaches associated with the common cold. It is particularly useful for headaches that feel congestive, throbbing, or are triggered by sinus congestion. Nux vomica can help reduce headache intensity and improve overall comfort.

4. **Supporting Digestion**: Nux vomica has properties that support digestive function. This can be beneficial during the common cold when digestion may be affected. By promoting healthy digestion, Nux vomica aids in overall wellness and may indirectly contribute to relieving cold symptoms.

5. **Individualized Treatment**: Homeopathy recognizes the importance of individualized treatment. While Nux vomica is commonly used for congestion and headaches, the response to homeopathic remedies may vary from person to person. It is recommended to follow the recommended dosage and consult with a qualified homeopath or healthcare professional for personalized guidance.

6. **Easy Administration**: Nux vomica is typically available in the form of small pellets. They can be dissolved under the tongue as directed on the product packaging. It is generally well-tolerated and suitable for adults and children.

7. **Complementary Approach**: Nux vomica can be used as a complementary approach alongside conventional medical treatment. It is important to

consult with a healthcare professional before using homeopathic remedies to ensure compatibility with other medications or treatments.

8. **Precautions**: Although Nux vomica is generally considered safe, it is important to follow the recommended dosage and consult with a healthcare professional if you have specific health conditions, allergies, or concerns. If symptoms persist or worsen, seek medical advice.

While Nux vomica may provide relief from congestion and headaches during the common cold, it should not replace medical treatment or professional advice. It is important to consult with a healthcare professional for a comprehensive evaluation and appropriate treatment.

As we continue to explore homeopathic remedies for the common cold, we will uncover additional strategies to support your well-being and enhance your recovery process. Embrace the benefits of Nux vomica as a potential aid in alleviating congestion and headaches, promoting your overall health during the common cold.
[End of Section 3]

Chapter 14

Lifestyle Practices for Cold Prevention

Section 1: Hand Hygiene - Proper Handwashing
Techniques

Hand hygiene, particularly proper handwashing techniques, plays a crucial role in preventing the spread of the common cold. In this section, we will explore the importance of hand hygiene and provide guidelines for proper handwashing techniques.

1. **Significance of Hand Hygiene:** Proper hand hygiene is one of the most effective ways to prevent the transmission of cold viruses. The common cold is primarily spread through contact with contaminated surfaces or respiratory droplets. Regular handwashing helps eliminate viruses and bacteria that may be present on the hands, reducing the risk of infection.

2. **Duration of Handwashing:** To ensure thorough cleaning, it is recommended to wash your hands for

at least 20 seconds. This duration allows sufficient time to lather, scrub, and rinse the hands effectively.

3. **Handwashing Steps**: Follow these steps to practice proper handwashing techniques:

a. Wet your hands with clean, running water (warm or cold). b. Apply soap and lather well, covering all surfaces of the hands, including the back, between fingers, and under nails. c. Scrub your hands vigorously for at least 20 seconds. You can use a timer or sing a song to ensure adequate duration. d. Pay attention to the fingertips, thumbs, and wrists during the scrubbing process. e. Rinse your hands thoroughly under clean, running water, ensuring all soap is removed. f. Dry your hands using a clean towel or air dry them. If using a towel, consider using a disposable one or a designated hand towel that is regularly cleaned.

4. **Hand Sanitizers**: In situations where soap and water are not readily available, alcohol-based hand sanitizers can be used as an alternative. Choose a hand sanitizer with at least 60% alcohol content and follow the instructions for proper application. However, it's important to note that hand sanitizers are not as effective as handwashing when hands are visibly dirty or greasy.

5. **Key Moments for Handwashing**: Practice handwashing at key moments, including:

a. Before and after preparing food b. Before eating or handling food c. After using the restroom d. After blowing your nose, coughing, or sneezing e. After touching surfaces in public areas (e.g., doorknobs, handrails) f. After caring for someone who is sick

6. **Role Modeling and Education**: Promote proper hand hygiene within your household and community by being a role model. Educate family members, especially children, about the importance

of handwashing and guide them in adopting proper handwashing techniques.

7. **Additional Hygiene Practices**: While handwashing is vital, it should be complemented by other hygiene practices, including covering your mouth and nose with a tissue or elbow when coughing or sneezing, avoiding close contact with sick individuals, and regularly disinfecting frequently touched surfaces.

Remember, hand hygiene is an essential component of cold prevention, but it should be practiced alongside other preventive measures, such as maintaining a healthy lifestyle and receiving recommended vaccinations.

As we continue to explore lifestyle practices for cold prevention, we will uncover additional strategies to promote a healthy and cold-free environment. Embrace the importance of proper hand hygiene and make it a regular habit in your daily routine to protect yourself and others from the common cold.

[End of Section 1]

Section 2: Avoiding Close Contact with Sick Individuals

Avoiding close contact with sick individuals is an essential practice for preventing the spread of the common cold. In this section, we will explore the significance of avoiding close contact and provide guidance on how to implement this preventive measure effectively.

1. **Transmission of the Common Cold**: The common cold is primarily transmitted through

respiratory droplets when an infected person coughs, sneezes, or talks. These droplets can contain the cold virus and can be inhaled by individuals in close proximity. Avoiding close contact with sick individuals reduces the risk of exposure to these respiratory droplets.

2. **Maintain Physical Distance**: To minimize the risk of contracting the common cold, maintain a distance of at least 6 feet (about 2 meters) from individuals who are visibly sick or displaying cold-like symptoms. This distance helps reduce the chances of coming into direct contact with respiratory droplets.

3. **Social Etiquette**: Practice social etiquette by avoiding close contact, such as handshakes, hugs, or kisses, with individuals who are experiencing cold symptoms. Opt for non-contact greetings, such as waving or nodding, as a respectful and preventive measure.

4. **Public Spaces and Crowded Areas**: Exercise caution in public spaces and crowded areas, where the risk of exposure to sick individuals may be higher. If possible, avoid densely populated environments or situations where close contact is difficult to avoid.

5. **Stay Home When Sick**: If you are experiencing cold symptoms, be considerate of others and stay home to prevent spreading the virus. By avoiding close contact with others, you can help break the chain of transmission and protect the health of those around you.

6. **Encourage Sick Individuals to Seek Medical Attention**: If you notice someone displaying cold symptoms, encourage them to seek medical attention and stay home until they recover. By

promoting responsible behavior, you can contribute to the overall well-being of your community.

7. **Practicing Good Respiratory Hygiene**: In addition to avoiding close contact with sick individuals, encourage proper respiratory hygiene among those who are sick. Encourage them to cover their mouth and nose with a tissue or their elbow when coughing or sneezing to prevent the spread of respiratory droplets.

8. **Be Mindful of Vulnerable Individuals**: Take extra precautions when interacting with vulnerable individuals, such as the elderly or those with compromised immune systems. These individuals are at higher risk of severe illness from the common cold. Minimizing close contact and practicing good respiratory hygiene is particularly crucial in these situations.

Remember, while avoiding close contact with sick individuals is an effective preventive measure, it should be practiced alongside other preventive measures, such as proper hand hygiene, respiratory etiquette, and maintaining a healthy lifestyle.

As we continue to explore lifestyle practices for cold prevention, we will uncover additional strategies to promote a healthy and cold-free environment. Embrace the importance of avoiding close contact with sick individuals as a responsible and proactive step in protecting yourself and others from the common cold.

[End of Section 2]

Section 3: Strengthening Overall Health

Strengthening overall health is a key component in preventing the common cold. In this section, we will explore the significance of maintaining a healthy lifestyle and provide guidance on how to strengthen your overall health to reduce the risk of colds.

1. **Balanced Diet**: A well-balanced diet rich in fruits, vegetables, whole grains, and lean proteins provides essential nutrients that support a healthy immune system. Include a variety of colorful fruits and vegetables in your meals to ensure an adequate intake of vitamins, minerals, and antioxidants.

2. **Hydration**: Staying hydrated is essential for maintaining overall health. Drink plenty of fluids, such as water, herbal teas, and clear broths, to keep your body hydrated and support optimal immune function.

3. **Regular Exercise**: Engaging in regular physical activity boosts overall health and strengthens the immune system. Aim for at least 150 minutes of moderate-intensity aerobic exercise or 75 minutes of vigorous-intensity exercise per week. Choose activities you enjoy, such as walking, cycling, or dancing, to make exercise a sustainable part of your routine.

4. **Adequate Sleep**: Quality sleep plays a vital role in maintaining a robust immune system. Aim for 7-9 hours of restful sleep each night to support your body's natural defense mechanisms and enhance overall health.

5. **Stress Management**: Chronic stress weakens the immune system, making you more susceptible to infections like the common cold. Practice stress management techniques, such as mindfulness meditation, deep breathing exercises, or engaging in

hobbies, to reduce stress levels and promote overall well-being.

6. **Avoid Smoking and Limit Alcohol**: Smoking damages the respiratory system and weakens the immune system, making you more susceptible to respiratory infections. Avoid smoking and limit alcohol consumption, as excessive alcohol intake can impair immune function. Opt for healthier alternatives and seek support if you need assistance in quitting smoking or managing alcohol consumption.

7. **Regular Vaccinations**: Stay up-to-date with recommended vaccinations, such as the flu vaccine, to protect against common viral infections. Consult with your healthcare provider to determine which vaccines are appropriate for you based on your age, medical history, and current recommendations.

8. **Personal Hygiene**: Maintain good personal hygiene practices, such as regularly washing your hands with soap and water, using hand sanitizers when necessary, and avoiding touching your face, nose, and eyes with unwashed hands. These practices help prevent the transmission of viruses and reduce the risk of contracting the common cold.

Remember, strengthening overall health is a lifelong commitment that goes beyond preventing the common cold. By adopting healthy lifestyle practices, you enhance your overall well-being and improve your body's ability to fight off infections.

As we conclude our exploration of lifestyle practices for cold prevention, embrace the importance of maintaining a healthy lifestyle and take proactive steps to strengthen your overall health. By doing so, you not only reduce the risk of the common cold but also enjoy numerous benefits for your well-being. [End of section 3]

Chapter 15

Traditional Remedies from Around the World

Section 1: Ayurvedic Remedies - Turmeric and Holy Basil

Ayurveda, an ancient system of medicine from India, offers a wealth of traditional remedies for various ailments, including the common cold. In this section, we will explore two Ayurvedic remedies, turmeric and holy basil, and their potential benefits in combating the common cold.

1. **Turmeric**: Turmeric, a vibrant yellow spice commonly used in Ayurvedic medicine, possesses powerful anti-inflammatory and antioxidant properties. It contains a compound called curcumin, which provides numerous health benefits. When it comes to the common cold, turmeric can be particularly beneficial due to its immune-boosting and symptom-relieving properties.

a. Immune-Boosting Properties: Turmeric supports the immune system by enhancing the activity of immune cells and promoting their response to pathogens. This can help strengthen the body's defense against cold viruses and reduce the severity and duration of symptoms.

b. Anti-inflammatory Action: The anti-inflammatory properties of turmeric can help alleviate symptoms such as nasal congestion, sore throat, and cough. It can help reduce inflammation in the respiratory tract, ease breathing difficulties, and provide relief from discomfort.

c. Ways to Incorporate Turmeric: Turmeric can be consumed as a spice in cooking or taken as a supplement. Consider adding turmeric powder to soups, stews, teas, or golden milk (a warm beverage made with turmeric, milk, and other spices) to enjoy its potential benefits during the common cold.

2. **Holy Basil**: Holy basil, also known as Tulsi, is a sacred herb in Ayurveda and is revered for its medicinal properties. It has been traditionally used to support respiratory health and alleviate cold symptoms. Holy basil is known for its antibacterial, antiviral, and immunomodulatory properties, making it a valuable herb for combating the common cold.

a. Respiratory Health Support: Holy basil has a soothing effect on the respiratory system and helps alleviate symptoms such as cough, congestion, and bronchial irritation. It acts as an expectorant, helping to expel phlegm and promote clearer breathing.

b. Immune-Boosting Effects: Holy basil boosts immune function, enhancing the body's natural defense mechanisms against viral infections like the common cold. It helps strengthen the immune response and supports overall respiratory health.

c. Ways to Use Holy Basil: Holy basil leaves can be used to prepare tea by steeping them in hot water for 5-10 minutes.

Adding honey and lemon can enhance the taste and provide additional soothing properties. Sip on holy basil tea several times a day to experience its potential benefits.

Both turmeric and holy basil are widely available and can be incorporated into your daily routine as part of a holistic approach to combating the common cold. However, it is important to note that individual responses may vary, and consulting with an Ayurvedic practitioner or healthcare professional is advisable, especially if you have specific health conditions, allergies, or concerns.

As we explore traditional remedies from around the world, we will uncover additional strategies to support your well-being and enhance your recovery process. Embrace the wisdom of Ayurveda and consider incorporating turmeric and holy basil into your routine to potentially alleviate symptoms and promote your overall health during the common cold.
[End of Section 1]

Section 2: Chinese Herbal Medicine - Astragalus and Honeysuckle

Chinese herbal medicine offers a rich tradition of remedies for various health conditions, including the common cold. In this section, we will explore two Chinese herbal remedies, astragalus and honeysuckle, and their potential benefits in combating the common cold.

1. **Astragalus:** Astragalus, also known as Huang Qi, is a popular herb in Traditional Chinese Medicine (TCM) with a long history of use for immune system support and respiratory health. It is believed

to enhance the body's defensive energy, known as Qi, and strengthen overall vitality.

a. **Immune System Support**: Astragalus is known for its immune-boosting properties. It helps stimulate and strengthen the immune system, making it more effective in fighting off viral infections like the common cold. By enhancing immune function, astragalus may help reduce the severity and duration of cold symptoms.

b. **Respiratory Health Benefits**: Astragalus is believed to have positive effects on respiratory health. It can help alleviate symptoms such as cough, sore throat, and nasal congestion by reducing inflammation and promoting respiratory comfort.

c. **Ways to Use Astragalus**: Astragalus is often prepared as a decoction or tea by boiling the dried root slices in water. It can also be found in supplement form, such as capsules or extracts. Follow the recommended dosage and consult with a TCM practitioner or healthcare professional for personalized guidance.

2. **Honeysuckle**: Honeysuckle, known as Jin Yin Hua in TCM, has been used for centuries in Chinese herbal medicine to address various ailments, including cold-related symptoms. It is valued for its antimicrobial, anti-inflammatory, and detoxifying properties.

a. **Antiviral and Antibacterial Effects**: Honeysuckle possesses potent antiviral and antibacterial properties, which can help combat cold viruses and reduce the risk of secondary infections. It may assist in inhibiting the growth of bacteria and viruses in the respiratory system.

b. **Soothing Inflammation**: Honeysuckle has anti-inflammatory effects that can help soothe inflamed respiratory tissues. It may help alleviate symptoms such as sore throat, cough, and nasal congestion, providing relief and promoting respiratory comfort.

c. **Ways to Use Honeysuckle**: Honeysuckle can be prepared as a herbal tea by steeping the dried flowers in hot water for 10-15 minutes. Adding other herbs like chrysanthemum or mint can enhance its benefits and flavor. Consult with a TCM practitioner or healthcare professional for proper usage and dosage.

Both astragalus and honeysuckle are important herbs in Chinese herbal medicine and can be valuable additions to your cold-fighting arsenal. However, it is essential to consult with a TCM practitioner or healthcare professional before using these remedies, especially if you have specific health conditions, allergies, or concerns.

As we explore traditional remedies from around the world, we will uncover additional strategies to support your well-being and enhance your recovery process. Embrace the wisdom of Chinese herbal medicine and consider incorporating astragalus and honeysuckle into your routine to potentially alleviate symptoms and promote your overall health during the common cold.
[End of Section 2]

Section 3: Indigenous Remedies - Echinacea and Elderberry

Indigenous cultures around the world have a rich tradition of using natural remedies to support health and well-being. In this section, we will explore two popular indigenous remedies, echinacea and elderberry, known for their potential benefits in combating the common cold.

1. **Echinacea**: Echinacea, a flowering plant native to North America, has long been used by indigenous

peoples for its immune-boosting properties. It is believed to enhance the activity of immune cells, supporting the body's defense against infections like the common cold.

a. **Immune-Enhancing Properties**: Echinacea is known to stimulate the immune system by increasing the production and activity of immune cells. It can help strengthen the body's natural defenses and reduce the severity and duration of cold symptoms.

b. **Anti-inflammatory Effects**: Echinacea also possesses anti-inflammatory properties, which can help alleviate symptoms such as sore throat, nasal congestion, and cough. By reducing inflammation, it promotes respiratory comfort and overall well-being.

c. **Forms and Usage**: Echinacea is available in various forms, including teas, tinctures, capsules, and extracts. Follow the recommended dosage and consult with a healthcare professional for proper usage and dosage based on your specific needs.

2. **Elderberry**: Elderberry, derived from the elder tree, has a long history of use in indigenous cultures for its immune-boosting and antiviral properties. It is rich in antioxidants and flavonoids that help support immune function.

a. **Immune-Boosting Effects**: Elderberry stimulates the production of cytokines, which are important for immune regulation. It can help enhance the body's natural defenses, reduce the severity of cold symptoms, and support a quicker recovery.

b. **Antiviral Properties**: Elderberry contains compounds that inhibit the replication of viruses, including those responsible for the common cold. It may help reduce the duration and intensity of symptoms by targeting the viruses causing the illness.

c. **Forms and Usage**: Elderberry can be consumed as syrups, extracts, capsules, or teas. Follow the recommended dosage and consult with a healthcare professional for proper usage and dosage based on your specific needs. Indigenous remedies like echinacea and elderberry offer valuable contributions to natural cold-fighting strategies. However, it is important to note that individual responses may vary, and consulting with a healthcare professional is advisable, especially if you have specific health conditions, allergies, or concerns.

As we explore indigenous remedies for the common cold, we embrace the wisdom and traditions of different cultures. Incorporating echinacea and elderberry into your routine may potentially support your immune system and aid in relieving common cold symptoms.
[End of Section 3]

Chapter 16

Natural Remedies for Children

Section 1: Caring for a Child with a Cold

When children catch a cold, it can be challenging for both them and their parents. In this section, we will explore natural remedies and practices to help care for a child with a cold, promoting their comfort and supporting their recovery.

1. **Provide Comfort and Rest:** Ensure that your child gets plenty of rest to aid in their recovery. Create a comfortable environment by adjusting the room temperature, using a humidifier to add moisture to the air, and providing cozy bedding.

2. **Encourage Hydration:** Proper hydration is crucial for children with colds, as it helps soothe sore throats, loosen congestion, and prevent dehydration. Offer fluids like water, herbal teas,

warm broths, or diluted fruit juices to keep them hydrated throughout the day.

3. **Nasal Saline Drops or Spray**: Nasal saline drops or sprays can help relieve nasal congestion in children. These natural solutions help moisten and loosen mucus, making it easier for your child to breathe. Use a bulb syringe or nasal aspirator to gently clear their nasal passages if needed.

4. **Honey for Cough Relief**: For children above the age of one, honey can be a natural remedy to soothe coughs. Add a teaspoon of honey to warm water or herbal tea. However, it is essential not to give honey to children under one year of age due to the risk of infant botulism.

5. **Steam Therapy**: Steam therapy can provide relief from congestion and coughs. Create a steamy environment in the bathroom by running a hot shower and sitting with your child in the steam-filled room for a few minutes. Ensure they are supervised to avoid any accidents with hot water or steam.

6. **Warm Liquids**: Offer warm liquids like herbal teas or warm water with a squeeze of lemon to soothe sore throats and promote hydration. Avoid giving hot beverages to children to prevent burns.

7. **Nutritious Foods**: Provide nourishing foods that are easy to eat and digest, such as soups, warm porridge, or soft fruits. Focus on nutrient-rich options that support their immune system and overall well-being.

8. **Herbal Remedies for Children**: Certain herbs, such as chamomile or catnip, can be used in child-friendly doses to soothe discomfort and promote

relaxation. Consult with a pediatric herbalist or healthcare professional experienced in treating children for appropriate herbal remedies.

9. **Monitor Symptoms:** Keep a close eye on your child's symptoms and monitor their condition. If symptoms worsen or persist for an extended period, consult a pediatrician or healthcare professional for further evaluation and guidance.

10. **Maintain Good Hygiene Practices:** Teach and reinforce good hygiene practices to your child, such as proper handwashing techniques, covering their mouth and nose with a tissue or elbow when coughing or sneezing, and avoiding close contact with others to prevent the spread of the cold virus.

Remember, every child is unique, and their response to remedies may vary. If you have any concerns or your child has underlying health conditions, it is advisable to consult with a pediatrician or healthcare professional before using natural remedies.

As we explore natural remedies for children with colds, we aim to provide comfort and support their well-being. By incorporating these practices, you can help your child through the discomfort of a cold and promote their speedy recovery.

[End of Section 1]

Section 2: Age-Appropriate Remedies and Precautions

When caring for a child with a cold, it is essential to consider age-appropriate remedies and take necessary precautions to ensure their safety and well-being. In this section, we will explore remedies and precautions specific to different age groups.

1. **Infants (Under 1 Year):** a. Ensure adequate hydration by breastfeeding or bottle-feeding frequently. Avoid giving water or other fluids unless advised by a healthcare professional. b. Use a nasal bulb syringe or saline drops to gently clear nasal congestion. c. Elevate the head of the crib or bassinet slightly to ease breathing. d. Consult a pediatrician before using any herbal remedies, cough syrups, or over-the-counter medications.

2. **Toddlers (1-3 Years):** a. Encourage hydration through sips of water, herbal teas, or diluted fruit juices. b. Use saline nasal drops or sprays to relieve nasal congestion. c. Offer age-appropriate honey-based remedies to soothe coughs. d. Provide simple and nutritious foods that are easy to eat and digest. e. Use child-friendly vapor rubs or chest rubs to relieve congestion, following the product's instructions. f. Maintain good hand hygiene and teach proper handwashing techniques.

3. **Preschoolers (3-5 Years):** a. Continue to prioritize hydration through water, herbal teas, and diluted fruit juices. b. Teach and encourage proper handwashing techniques. c. Offer warm soups, broths, and nourishing foods to support their immune system. d. Consider age-appropriate herbal remedies, such as chamomile tea, to promote relaxation and relieve symptoms. e. Use saline nasal drops or sprays and teach your child how to blow their nose gently. f. Provide a humidifier in their bedroom to add moisture to the air.

4. **School-Age Children (6-12 Years):** a. Encourage self-care practices, such as blowing their nose, proper handwashing, and covering their mouth when coughing or sneezing. b. Offer warm liquids, like herbal teas or warm water with lemon, to soothe sore throats and promote hydration. c. Teach the importance of rest and ensure they have a comfortable sleeping environment. d. Consider natural throat lozenges or cough drops appropriate for their age. e. Support their immune system with a balanced diet rich in fruits, vegetables, and whole grains. f. Engage in age-appropriate conversations about the importance of good hygiene practices to prevent the spread of germs.

Remember to consult with a pediatrician or healthcare professional before using any new remedies or over-the-counter medications, especially for young children. Each child is unique, and their individual needs should be taken into consideration.

By using age-appropriate remedies and precautions, you can effectively support your child's recovery from a cold while ensuring their safety and well-being.
[End of Section 2]

Chapter 17

Seeking Medical Help

Section: When to Consult a Healthcare Professional

While most common colds can be managed at home with natural remedies, there are instances when it is important to seek medical help. In this section, we will discuss situations in which consulting a healthcare professional is recommended when dealing with a common cold.

1. **High Fever:** If your child, or even yourself, has a persistent high fever (typically over 100.4°F or 38°C), it is advisable to seek medical attention. A high fever accompanied by other concerning symptoms may indicate a more severe infection that requires medical evaluation.

2. **Difficulty Breathing:** If you or your child experience difficulty breathing, rapid or shallow breathing, or wheezing, it is essential to seek

immediate medical attention. These symptoms may indicate a more serious respiratory condition that needs prompt evaluation and treatment.

3. **Severe or Prolonged Symptoms**: If cold symptoms persist or worsen after a week or so, or if they become significantly severe, it is advisable to consult a healthcare professional. This is especially important if symptoms include persistent coughing, severe sore throat, persistent headache, earache, or chest pain.

4. **Underlying Health Conditions**: If you or your child have underlying health conditions, such as asthma, weakened immune system, or chronic respiratory disorders, it is important to consult a healthcare professional. They can provide appropriate guidance and ensure that the cold does not exacerbate any existing health issues.

5. **Persistent Ear Pain or Drainage**: If you or your child experience persistent ear pain or drainage from the ears, it may indicate an ear infection or other complications. Seeking medical advice is important to prevent any further complications or potential damage to the ears.

6. **Concerns with Infant or Young Child**: If your infant or young child (under 3 months old) shows signs of a cold, it is advisable to consult a healthcare professional. Babies at this age are more vulnerable to complications from respiratory infections and may require closer monitoring and evaluation.

7. **Worsening Overall Condition**: If you or your child's overall condition continues to deteriorate despite home remedies and self-care measures, it is crucial to seek medical help. This includes

symptoms like persistent fatigue, dehydration, lethargy, or signs of dehydration.
Remember, the above situations serve as general guidelines, and it is always important to trust your instincts as a caregiver. If you have any concerns about your or your child's health, it is best to seek medical advice to ensure proper evaluation and appropriate treatment.

As we conclude our exploration of seeking medical help for the common cold, remember that healthcare professionals are there to support and guide you in managing your health and well-being. By seeking their expertise when needed, you can ensure the best possible care for yourself or your loved ones.
[End of Section 1]

Section 2: Understanding the Difference Between a Cold and the Flu

It can sometimes be challenging to differentiate between a common cold and the flu (influenza) since they share similar symptoms. However, understanding the differences can help you make informed decisions regarding your health. In this section, we will explore the distinctions between a cold and the flu.

1. Onset and Duration:
    - Cold: Symptoms of a cold typically develop gradually over a few days and tend to last for about a week, sometimes slightly longer.
    - Flu: Influenza symptoms usually have a sudden onset and can be more severe than

a cold. The flu typically lasts for about one to two weeks, with lingering fatigue and weakness.

2. Symptoms:
    - Cold: Common cold symptoms often include a runny or stuffy nose, sneezing, sore throat, and mild to moderate cough. Mild fatigue and a low-grade fever may occur in some cases.
    - Flu: Influenza symptoms are more intense and may include high fever (above 100.4°F or 38°C), body aches, headache, severe fatigue, dry cough, sore throat, and nasal congestion.
3. Fatigue and Weakness:
    - Cold: Fatigue and weakness with a cold are usually mild and do not significantly impact daily activities.
    - Flu: Fatigue and weakness with the flu can be severe and can last for several weeks, making it difficult to carry out normal routines.
4. Body Aches and Headaches:
    - Cold: Body aches and headaches associated with a cold are generally mild and localized.
    - Flu: Influenza often causes more pronounced body aches, joint pain, and headaches that can be severe and widespread.
5. Complications:
    - Cold: Colds generally do not lead to serious health complications. However, they can occasionally exacerbate existing respiratory

conditions, such as asthma or chronic bronchitis.

- **Flu**: The flu can lead to complications, especially in high-risk individuals such as young children, older adults, pregnant women, and those with weakened immune systems. These complications may include pneumonia, sinus infections, ear infections, or worsening of chronic medical conditions.

6. **Seasonal Patterns**:

- Cold: Colds can occur at any time throughout the year, although they are more prevalent during colder months.
- Flu: Influenza typically has a seasonal pattern, with higher activity during the fall and winter months.

It's important to note that this information serves as a general guide, and individual experiences may vary. If you have concerns about your symptoms or are unsure about your condition, it is advisable to consult a healthcare professional for proper evaluation and guidance.

By understanding the differences between a cold and the flu, you can better assess your symptoms and take appropriate measures to manage your health effectively. [End of section 2]

Chapter 18

Myths and Misconceptions about Colds

Section 1: Debunking Common Cold Myths

The common cold is a widely experienced ailment, and over time, various myths and misconceptions have emerged surrounding its causes, prevention, and treatment. In this section, we will debunk some common cold myths to provide accurate information and promote a better understanding of this prevalent condition.

1. **Myth a.**: Cold Weather Causes Colds: Fact: Cold weather alone does not cause the common cold. Colds are caused by viruses, most commonly rhinoviruses, which are more prevalent during colder months. However, the primary factor in contracting a cold is exposure to the virus, not the temperature.

2. **Myth b.**: Going Outside with Wet Hair Causes Colds: Fact: The idea that going outside with wet

hair leads to a cold is a common misconception. Colds are caused by viruses, not by external factors such as wet hair. While exposure to cold temperatures may temporarily lower your body's defenses, it does not directly cause a cold.

3. **Myth c.**: Antibiotics Cure Colds: Fact: Antibiotics are not effective against the common cold. Colds are caused by viral infections, and antibiotics are specifically designed to treat bacterial infections. Taking antibiotics for a cold will not speed up recovery and may contribute to antibiotic resistance.

4. **Myth d.**: Vitamin C Prevents Colds: Fact: While vitamin C is important for a healthy immune system, there is no conclusive evidence that high-dose vitamin C prevents colds in the general population. However, maintaining a well-balanced diet rich in fruits and vegetables, including those high in vitamin C, supports overall immune health.

5. **Myth e.**: Being Cold or Wet Makes You Susceptible to Colds: Fact: Being cold or wet does not make you more susceptible to catching a cold. Colds are primarily spread through direct contact with infected respiratory secretions, such as coughs or sneezes, or by touching contaminated surfaces and then touching your face.

6. **Myth f.**: Exercise Causes Colds: Fact: Moderate exercise does not cause colds. In fact, regular exercise can boost the immune system and contribute to overall well-being. However, intense or prolonged exercise in cold weather may temporarily weaken the immune system, potentially increasing the risk of contracting a cold virus.

7. **Myth g.**: Chicken Soup Cures Colds: Fact: While chicken soup is often comforting and soothing during a cold, it does not cure the underlying viral infection. However, it can help alleviate symptoms and provide hydration and nourishment, making you feel better temporarily.

8. **Myth h.**: Colds Only Spread in Winter: Fact: While the common cold is more prevalent during colder months, it can occur at any time of the year. Viruses that cause colds are present throughout the year, and transmission can happen in any season, particularly in environments where people are in close contact.

It is important to rely on accurate information when it comes to understanding and managing the common cold. By debunking these myths, we can make informed decisions about prevention, treatment, and overall well-being.

As we conclude this section on debunking common cold myths, remember to seek reliable sources and consult healthcare professionals for accurate information regarding the common cold and other health-related matters.

[End of Section 1]

Section 2: Differentiating Facts from Fiction

In an era of readily available information, it is crucial to separate facts from fiction when it comes to understanding the common cold. Misinformation can lead to confusion and potentially ineffective or harmful practices. In this section, we will provide guidance on how to differentiate between facts and fiction regarding the common cold.

1. Reliable Sources:
   - Fact: Rely on credible sources of information such as reputable medical websites, healthcare organizations, and trusted healthcare professionals. These sources undergo rigorous review processes and provide evidence-based information.
   - Fiction: Be cautious of information from unofficial websites, social media posts, or unverified sources. While the internet can be a helpful resource, misinformation can easily spread. Look for information that is supported by scientific research and backed by credible institutions.

2. Scientific Research:
   - Fact: Scientific research plays a crucial role in understanding diseases and treatments. Look for studies published in reputable scientific journals. Peer-reviewed research is more likely to provide reliable information.
   - Fiction: Avoid basing decisions solely on anecdotal evidence or personal testimonials. While individual experiences are valuable, they may not reflect general trends or reliable scientific evidence.

3. Consensus Among Experts:
   - Fact: Consensus among experts within the medical and scientific community is an important factor in establishing reliable

information. Look for areas of agreement among multiple experts in the field.

- Fiction: Be cautious of isolated or fringe opinions that contradict established scientific consensus. Extraordinary claims should be scrutinized and validated by the broader scientific community.

4. **Evidence-Based Guidelines:**

- Fact: Evidence-based guidelines developed by reputable organizations, such as national health institutes, provide recommendations based on rigorous research and expert consensus. These guidelines are regularly updated to reflect the latest scientific evidence.
- Fiction: Avoid relying solely on personal opinions, alternative medicine claims, or unproven remedies that lack scientific backing. While alternative practices may have value in certain contexts, it is important to prioritize evidence-based approaches when it comes to your health.

5. **Personalized Advice:**

- Fact: Seek personalized advice from healthcare professionals who have a thorough understanding of your medical history and individual needs. They can provide tailored recommendations based on reliable information and your specific circumstances.
- Fiction: Be cautious of one-size-fits-all approaches or generalized advice that may not consider your unique situation. Each person's health and circumstances are

different, and individualized advice is essential for optimal care.
By following these guidelines and being critical of the information you encounter, you can better navigate the vast amount of information available and make informed decisions regarding the common cold.

As we conclude this section on differentiating facts from fiction, remember to prioritize reliable sources, scientific evidence, consensus among experts, evidence-based guidelines, and personalized advice from healthcare professionals. By doing so, you can ensure that you have accurate information to effectively manage your health and well-being.
[End of Section 2]

Chapter 19

Coping with Cold-Related Complications

Section 1: Sinusitis - Symptoms, Treatment, and Prevention

Sinusitis is a common complication that can arise from a cold, causing inflammation and infection of the sinus cavities. In this section, we will explore the symptoms, treatment options, and preventive measures for sinusitis.

1. **Symptoms of Sinusitis:**
   - Facial pain or pressure, particularly around the cheeks, eyes, and forehead.
   - Nasal congestion and difficulty breathing through the nose.
   - Thick yellow or green nasal discharge.
   - Reduced sense of smell and taste.
   - Coughing, especially at night.

- Headache, often worsened by bending forward or lying down.
- Fatigue and a general feeling of malaise.

2. **Treatment Options:**
   - Rest and Hydration: Get plenty of rest and stay hydrated to support your body's healing process.
   - Nasal Irrigation: Use saline nasal sprays or a neti pot to flush out the sinuses and relieve congestion.
   - Warm Compresses: Apply warm compresses to the face to alleviate pain and promote sinus drainage.
   - Pain Relief: Over-the-counter pain relievers like acetaminophen or ibuprofen can help reduce facial pain and headache.
   - Decongestants: Short-term use of oral or nasal decongestants may provide temporary relief from nasal congestion. However, consult a healthcare professional before using them, especially if you have underlying health conditions.
   - Antibiotics: If sinusitis is bacterial in nature or becomes chronic, a healthcare professional may prescribe antibiotics to treat the infection.
   - Corticosteroids: In some cases, corticosteroid nasal sprays may be recommended to reduce inflammation and promote healing.

3. **Preventive Measures:**
   - Manage Nasal Congestion: Address nasal congestion promptly by using saline nasal sprays or decongestants as directed.

- Maintain Good Hygiene: Practice proper hand hygiene, such as frequent handwashing, to reduce the risk of spreading germs.
- Stay Hydrated: Drink plenty of fluids to keep your nasal passages hydrated and facilitate mucus drainage.
- Avoid Irritants: Minimize exposure to environmental irritants, such as smoke and pollutants, which can aggravate sinusitis symptoms.
- Use Humidifiers: Use a humidifier or vaporizer to add moisture to the air, particularly during dry conditions or in heated environments.
- Quit Smoking: If you smoke, consider quitting as smoking can exacerbate sinusitis symptoms and delay healing.
- Allergy Management: If you have allergies, effectively manage them to reduce the risk of sinusitis. Consult an allergist for appropriate allergy management strategies.

It is important to consult a healthcare professional if your symptoms worsen or persist despite self-care measures or if you suspect a bacterial infection. They can provide an accurate diagnosis and recommend the most appropriate treatment plan for your specific condition.

As we conclude this section on sinusitis, remember that prompt and proper management can help alleviate symptoms and support healing. By practicing preventive measures and seeking timely medical attention when needed, you can cope with and effectively address

complications associated with the common cold.
[End of Section 1]

Section 2: Bronchitis - Managing Respiratory Inflammation

Bronchitis is a respiratory condition characterized by inflammation of the bronchial tubes, often resulting from a cold or viral infection. In this section, we will discuss strategies for managing respiratory inflammation associated with bronchitis.

1. Symptoms of Bronchitis:
   - Persistent cough that may produce mucus or phlegm.
   - Chest discomfort or tightness.
   - Shortness of breath or wheezing.
   - Fatigue and general feeling of malaise.
   - Mild fever or chills in some cases.
2. Treatment Options:
   - Rest and Hydration: Get plenty of rest to allow your body to heal. Drink ample fluids to stay hydrated and help loosen mucus.
   - Cough Suppressants: Over-the-counter cough suppressants can provide temporary relief from persistent coughing. However, consult a healthcare professional before using them, especially if you have underlying health conditions.
   - Expectorants: Expectorant medications help thin and loosen mucus, making it easier to cough up. Follow the instructions on the

label or consult a healthcare professional for appropriate use.

- Inhalation Therapy: Steam inhalation or using a humidifier can help moisturize and soothe the airways, reducing coughing and promoting easier breathing.
- Bronchodilators: If bronchitis causes significant breathing difficulties or wheezing, a healthcare professional may prescribe bronchodilator medications to relax and open the airways.
- Antibiotics: Most cases of bronchitis are caused by viruses and do not require antibiotics. However, if bacterial infection is suspected or if you have underlying health conditions, antibiotics may be prescribed.

3. **Self-Care Measures:**

- Avoid Irritants: Minimize exposure to irritants such as smoke, strong chemicals, and pollutants, which can further irritate the bronchial tubes.
- Warm Fluids: Sip on warm fluids like herbal teas or warm water with honey and lemon to soothe the throat and help thin mucus.
- Steam Therapy: Take warm showers or create a steamy environment by filling a bowl with hot water and inhaling the steam to ease congestion and loosen mucus.
- Maintain Good Indoor Air Quality: Keep indoor spaces well-ventilated and clean to reduce potential triggers for respiratory irritation.

- Use a Humidifier: A humidifier or vaporizer can add moisture to the air, relieving dryness and promoting easier breathing.
- Avoid Cough Suppressants for Productive Cough: If your cough produces mucus or phlegm, avoid using cough suppressants, as coughing helps clear the airways.

4. Follow Medical Advice:

- If your symptoms worsen, persist for an extended period, or if you have underlying health conditions, seek medical attention promptly.
- Follow the prescribed treatment plan and take any medications as directed by a healthcare professional.
- Attend scheduled follow-up appointments to monitor your progress and ensure appropriate management of bronchitis.

Remember, bronchitis can range from acute to chronic, and proper management is essential for a full recovery. If you have concerns or your symptoms do not improve, it is important to consult a healthcare professional for a thorough evaluation and personalized treatment.

As we conclude this section on managing respiratory inflammation associated with bronchitis, be proactive in implementing self-care measures, following medical advice, and seeking timely medical attention when necessary. By effectively managing inflammation and supporting respiratory health, you can cope with the complications that may arise from the common cold.
[End of Section 2]

Section 3: Ear Infections - Recognizing and Treating Them

Ear infections can occur as a complication of a cold, especially in children. In this section, we will discuss how to recognize the symptoms of ear infections and explore treatment options.

1. Symptoms of Ear Infections:
    - Ear pain or discomfort, especially when lying down.
    - Tugging or pulling at the ears, especially in infants and young children.
    - Fluid drainage from the ear(s).
    - Decreased hearing or difficulty hearing.
    - Irritability or fussiness, particularly in infants.
    - Fever, although it may not always be present.
2. Treatment Options:
    - Pain Relief: Over-the-counter pain relievers, such as acetaminophen or ibuprofen, can help alleviate ear pain. Follow the recommended dosage for age-appropriate use.
    - Warm Compresses: Applying a warm compress or heating pad to the affected ear can help alleviate pain and discomfort.
    - Ear Drops: Over-the-counter ear drops may provide relief from pain or help dry excessive moisture in the ears. Consult a healthcare professional or pharmacist for appropriate use.

- Antibiotics: If the ear infection is bacterial or if symptoms are severe, a healthcare professional may prescribe antibiotics. It is important to complete the full course of antibiotics as directed.

3. **Home Care Measures:**
   - Rest and Comfort: Ensure the affected person gets enough rest to aid in recovery. Provide a comfortable sleeping environment and prop their head up slightly to ease ear pressure.
   - Avoid Irritants: Keep the ears dry and avoid exposing them to irritants such as excessive water, smoke, or strong chemicals.
   - Nasal Saline Drops: If nasal congestion is present, use saline nasal drops or sprays to help relieve congestion and minimize the risk of spreading infection to the ears.
   - Follow-Up Care: Attend follow-up appointments as recommended by a healthcare professional to monitor the progress of the ear infection and ensure appropriate healing.

4. **When to Seek Medical Attention:**
   - If symptoms worsen or do not improve within a few days.
   - If severe pain or high fever develops.
   - If there is persistent fluid drainage from the ear.
   - If symptoms are accompanied by signs of hearing loss or balance problems.
   - If the affected person is an infant or has underlying health conditions.

It is important to consult a healthcare professional for an accurate diagnosis and appropriate treatment. They can examine the ears and determine the most effective course of action based on the individual's age, symptoms, and overall health.

As we conclude this section on recognizing and treating ear infections, remember to closely monitor symptoms, provide appropriate pain relief, practice home care measures, and seek medical attention when necessary. By promptly addressing ear infections, you can help alleviate discomfort and support the healing process.
[End of Section 3]

Chapter 20

Preventing Future Colds

Section 1: Building a Healthy Lifestyle to Prevent Illnesses

Preventing future colds involves adopting long-term strategies that promote a healthy lifestyle and support a robust immune system. In this section, we will explore various practices and habits you can incorporate into your life to reduce the risk of colds and other illnesses.

1. **Balanced Diet:**
    - Eat a nutrient-rich diet that includes a variety of fruits, vegetables, whole grains, lean proteins, and healthy fats.
    - Incorporate immune-boosting foods such as citrus fruits, berries, leafy greens, garlic, ginger, and yogurt containing live cultures.

- Stay adequately hydrated by drinking plenty of water throughout the day.

2. **Regular Exercise:**
   - Engage in regular physical activity to strengthen your immune system and overall health.
   - Aim for at least 150 minutes of moderate-intensity aerobic exercise or 75 minutes of vigorous-intensity exercise per week.
   - Choose activities you enjoy, such as brisk walking, cycling, swimming, or dancing.

3. **Quality Sleep:**
   - Prioritize sufficient and restful sleep to support immune function.
   - Aim for 7-9 hours of sleep per night, adjusting as needed based on individual requirements.
   - Establish a consistent sleep schedule and create a sleep-friendly environment with a comfortable mattress, dark curtains, and a quiet atmosphere.

4. **Stress Management:**
   - Chronic stress can weaken the immune system, making you more susceptible to illnesses like colds.
   - Practice stress management techniques such as deep breathing, meditation, yoga, or engaging in hobbies that promote relaxation.
   - Find healthy outlets for stress, such as exercise, spending time in nature, or connecting with loved ones.

5. **Hand Hygiene:**

- Wash your hands regularly with soap and water for at least 20 seconds, especially after coughing, sneezing, using the restroom, or being in public places.
- If soap and water are unavailable, use hand sanitizers containing at least 60% alcohol.
- Avoid touching your face, particularly your eyes, nose, and mouth, as it can facilitate the entry of viruses into your body.

6. Vaccinations:
- Stay up to date with recommended vaccinations, including the annual flu shot.
- Vaccinations help prevent certain viral infections and reduce the severity of illness if infection occurs.

7. Avoidance of Sick Individuals:
- Minimize close contact with individuals who have a cold or other respiratory infections.
- If you are sick, avoid close contact with others to prevent the spread of the virus.

8. Environmental Hygiene:
- Maintain cleanliness and good hygiene practices in your living spaces.
- Clean and disinfect frequently touched surfaces, such as doorknobs, light switches, and electronic devices.
- Ensure proper ventilation to improve air quality and minimize the concentration of airborne pathogens.

9. Smoking Cessation:
- If you smoke, quitting smoking is essential for improving your overall health and reducing the risk of respiratory infections, including colds.

- Seek support from healthcare professionals or smoking cessation programs to assist you in quitting.

By adopting these long-term strategies and incorporating them into your daily routine, you can strengthen your immune system and reduce the risk of future colds and other illnesses.

As we conclude this section on building a healthy lifestyle to prevent illnesses, remember that prevention is key. By making positive lifestyle choices, practicing good hygiene, and prioritizing your overall well-being, you can minimize your susceptibility to colds and promote long-term health. [End of section 1]

Conclusion

Embracing the Wisdom of Old-Fashioned Remedies

In the fast-paced modern world, where we are surrounded by advanced medical technologies and pharmaceutical options, it's easy to overlook the wisdom of old-fashioned home remedies. However, as we have explored in this book, there is immense value in embracing these traditional remedies when it comes to combating the common cold.

From understanding the common cold and its symptoms to exploring various remedies and preventive measures, we have delved into a wide range of topics. We have learned about the power of herbal remedies such as echinacea, ginger, elderberry, and peppermint in alleviating cold symptoms. We have explored the nourishing properties of healing soups and broths, the soothing effects of hot drinks and teas, and the benefits of steam inhalation and nasal irrigation.

But it doesn't stop there. We have also discussed the importance of rest, sleep, and creating a conducive environment for recovery. We have highlighted the significance of seeking medical help when necessary and debunked common myths and misconceptions surrounding colds. We have recognized the need to differentiate facts from fiction and provided guidance on recognizing and managing cold-related complications.

Furthermore, we have explored strategies for preventing future colds by building a healthy lifestyle. By focusing on balanced nutrition, regular exercise, quality sleep, stress management, hand hygiene, vaccinations, avoidance of sick individuals, environmental hygiene, and smoking cessation, we can reduce the risk of colds and enhance our overall well-being.

In embracing the wisdom of old-fashioned remedies, we tap into the rich traditions and knowledge passed down through generations. These remedies offer a holistic approach to healing, incorporating natural ingredients, time-tested practices, and self-care rituals that nourish our bodies and support our immune systems.

So, let us not overlook the power of these age-old remedies. Let us embrace the wisdom of our ancestors and integrate these practices into our lives. By doing so, we can find comfort, relief, and improved health when faced with the common cold.

Remember, each of us is unique, and what works for one person may vary for another. It's important to listen to your body, consult healthcare professionals when needed, and adapt these remedies to suit your individual needs.

As you journey forward, armed with the knowledge and insights shared in this book, may you find solace in the wisdom of old-fashioned home remedies and experience the amazing results they can bring in combating the common cold. Here's to a healthier, more resilient you!

Appendix

Useful Recipes and Resources

In this appendix, we provide you with a collection of useful recipes and additional resources to further explore the world of old-fashioned home remedies for the common cold.

1. Recipes:
    - Chicken Soup: A classic recipe for traditional cold-fighting chicken soup.
    - Vegetable Broth: A comforting and nourishing recipe for homemade vegetable broth.
    - Bone Broth: A nutrient-rich elixir made from simmering bones for an extended period.
    - Lemon and Honey Tea: A soothing and comforting beverage for relieving sore throat.
    - Turmeric Milk: A warm and anti-inflammatory elixir made with turmeric and milk.
    - Chamomile Tea: A calming herbal tea that helps soothe respiratory discomfort.
2. Additional Resources:

- Books: Explore the following books for more information on home remedies and natural health:
    - "The Complete Book of Home Remedies" by Dr. Vasant Lad and Dr. David Frawley
    - "Rosemary Gladstar's Herbal Recipes for Vibrant Health" by Rosemary Gladstar
    - "The Herbal Medicine-Maker's Handbook" by James Green
- **Websites**: Visit the following reputable websites for reliable information on natural remedies and health:
    - National Center for Complementary and Integrative Health (nccih.nih.gov)
    - Mayo Clinic (mayoclinic.org)
    - WebMD (webmd.com)
- **Traditional Medicine Practices**: Explore the rich traditions of Ayurveda, Traditional Chinese Medicine (TCM), and Indigenous healing practices for a deeper understanding of holistic health and remedies.

Remember to always consult healthcare professionals before trying any new remedies or if you have specific health concerns or conditions.

By exploring these recipes and resources, you can continue your journey into the world of old-fashioned home remedies, deepen your knowledge, and discover new ways to support your health and well-being.

Wishing you a healthy and fulfilling journey!

Glossary

In this glossary, you will find definitions of key terms and concepts related to old-fashioned home remedies and the common cold.

1. **Common Cold**: A viral infection primarily affecting the nose and throat, characterized by symptoms such as sneezing, congestion, runny nose, sore throat, and cough.

2. **Immune System**: The body's defense system against infections and diseases. It is composed of various cells, tissues, and organs that work together to identify and eliminate pathogens, including viruses.

3. **Herbal Remedies**: Natural remedies derived from plants, including herbs, flowers, roots, and leaves, that are used for their therapeutic properties. Examples include echinacea, ginger, and peppermint.

4. **Homeopathic Remedies**: Remedies based on the principle of "like cures like." Homeopathic treatments use highly diluted substances to stimulate the body's natural healing response.

5. **Saline Rinse**: A technique that involves using a saline solution to rinse the nasal passages, helping to relieve congestion, moisturize the nasal passages, and remove irritants.

6. **Steam Inhalation**: The practice of inhaling steam from hot water or herbal preparations to help open up the airways, soothe congestion, and relieve respiratory symptoms.

7. **Bronchitis**: Inflammation of the bronchial tubes, typically resulting from a viral infection. It is characterized by symptoms such as coughing, chest discomfort, and difficulty breathing.

8. **Sinusitis**: Inflammation of the sinuses, often caused by a viral or bacterial infection. It leads to symptoms such as facial pain or pressure, nasal congestion, and thick nasal discharge.

9. **Ear Infection**: Infection or inflammation of the middle ear, commonly caused by viral or bacterial infections. It is characterized by symptoms such as ear pain, fluid drainage, and reduced hearing.

10. **Immune Booster**: Substances or practices that support and enhance the immune system's function, helping to protect against infections and diseases.

11. **Elixir**: A concentrated liquid containing medicinal or therapeutic properties, often used to promote health and well-being.

12. **Peer-Reviewed Research**: Research studies that have undergone a rigorous evaluation process by experts in the field before publication. This process ensures the quality and validity of the research.

13. **Evidence-Based**: Information or practices that are supported by scientific research and empirical evidence, ensuring their effectiveness and reliability.

14. **Nasal Irrigation**: The process of flushing the nasal passages with a saline solution to cleanse and moisturize the nasal cavities, providing relief from congestion and improving nasal health.

15. **Antioxidant**: Substances that help protect the body against oxidative stress and damage caused by harmful free radicals, which can contribute to various health conditions.
16. **Adaptogen**: Natural substances that help the body adapt and cope with stress, supporting overall well-being and promoting homeostasis.
17. **Immune Support**: Practices, habits, and remedies that boost and strengthen the immune system's ability to fight off infections and maintain optimal health.
18. **Respiratory Inflammation**: Inflammation of the respiratory system, which includes the nasal passages, throat, bronchial tubes, and lungs. It can result from various factors, including infections and irritants.
19. **Wellness**: The state of overall well-being, encompassing physical, mental, and emotional health.
20. **Holistic Health**: A comprehensive approach to health and well-being that considers the interplay between physical, mental, emotional, and spiritual aspects of an individual's life.

This glossary provides a reference for key terms used throughout the book, helping to enhance your understanding of the concepts discussed.
Note: The definitions provided are general and may not encompass all aspects or variations of each term.

Author, Stanley Hardy Mack
"Old Fashioned Home Remedies"
Copyrights 2023 All Rights Reserved

Thank you for considering leaving a review for "Old Fashioned Home Remedies - Common Cold" Combating with Amazing Results. Your thoughts and feedback are highly appreciated as they help me understand how the book has resonated with readers and how it can be improved in the future.

To leave a review, you can visit the platform where you purchased or accessed the book, such as an online bookstore or a review platform. Look for the book's page and navigate to the review section. There, you can share your thoughts, impressions, and overall rating for the book. You can also mention specific aspects that you found valuable or any suggestions you have for future editions.

Your review will not only provide valuable feedback for me as an author but also assist other potential readers in making an informed decision about the book. I truly appreciate your support and the time you take to share your thoughts.

Thank you once again for reading "Old Fashioned Home Remedies - Common Cold" Combating with Amazing Results. And for considering leaving a review. Your feedback is instrumental in shaping future projects and improving the overall reading experience.